D1457404

BELMONT UNIVERSITY LIBRARY
BELMONT UNIVERSITY
1900 BELMONT BLVD.
NASHVILLE, TN 37212

Case Studies for Manual Therapy

Note
Neither the publishers nor the authors will be liable for any loss
or damage of any nature occasioned to or suffered by any person
acting or refraining from acting as a result of reliance on the
material contained in this publication.

For Churchill Livingstone:

Commissioning editor: Mary Law
Project manager: Valerie Burgess
Project development editor: Valerie Bain
Project controller: Derek Robertson
Design direction: Judith Wright
Illustrator and designer: John Leech
Copy editor: Stephanie Pickering
Promotions manager: Hilary Brown

Case Studies for Manual Therapy

A Problem-Based Approach

Peter Spencer BSc MB BS PhD DO

Principal, London School of Osteopathy, London, UK

Foreword by
Dana J. Lawrence DC FICC

Editor, Journal of Manipulative and Physiological Therapeutics,
and Professor, Department of Chiropractic Practice,
National College of Chiropractic, Lombard, IL, USA

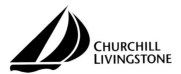

CHURCHILL
LIVINGSTONE

NEW YORK, EDINBURGH, LONDON, MADRID, MELBOURNE, SAN FRANCISCO AND TOKYO 1998

CHURCHILL LIVINGSTONE
Medical Division of Pearson Professional Limited

Distributed in the United States of America by Churchill
Livingstone Inc., 650 Avenue of the Americas, New York,
N.Y. 10011, and by associated companies, branches and
representatives throughout the world.

© Pearson Professional Limited 1998
⟯ is a registered trademark of Pearson Professional Ltd.

All rights reserved. No part of this publication may be
reproduced, stored in a retrieval system, or transmitted in any
form or by any means, electronic, mechanical, photocopying,
recording or otherwise, without either the prior permission of
the publishers (Churchill Livingstone, Robert Stevenson House,
1–3 Baxter's Place, Leith Walk, Edinburgh EH1 3AF), or a
licence permitting restricted copying in the United Kingdom
issued by the Copyright Licensing Agency Ltd, 90 Tottenham
Court Road, London W1P 9HE.

First published 1998

ISBN 0443 05696 X

British Library of Cataloguing in Publication Data
A catalogue record for this book is available from the British
Library.

Library of Congress Cataloging in Publication Data
A catalog record for this book is available from the Library of
Congress.

Note
Medical knowledge is constantly changing. As new information
becomes available, changes in treatment, procedures, equipment
and the use of drugs become necessary. The author and the
publishers have, as far as it is possible, taken care to ensure that
the information given in this text is accurate and up to date.
However, readers are strongly advised to confirm that the
information, especially with regard to drug usage, complies with
latest legislation and standards of practice.

The
publisher's
policy is to use
paper manufactured
from sustainable forests

Printed in Singapore

203932

BELMONT UNIVERSITY LIBRARY

RM
724
.S64
1998

ABC-3192

Contents

Foreword

Dr Peter Spencer's *Case Studies for Manual Therapy* is the book I wish I'd had years ago, when I was a student. Not only does it meet the needs of practitioners new to clinical practice but it also tackles the challenges posed by the development of problem-based learning programs.

As a faculty member at the National College of Chiropractic for the last 18 years, I have watched our approach to teaching and education undergo radical changes, leading to today's emphasis upon self-directed, problem-based education. When I first started my course of study at National, I was daunted by the huge amount of material I was expected to learn. As an undergraduate at Michigan State University, my typical course load per term was approximately 15 hours per week; at National, it was closer to 30 hours per week. Much of that time was spent sitting in class taking profuse amounts of notes, which I would later return to so that I could study them for the tests that were so frequently scheduled. A great deal of the material I studied was based upon didactic lectures, in which fact after fact was presented. I thought that memorizing these facts would help make me a good doctor; indeed, many of my classmates felt the same. We were very good at memorization and we surely passed our tests.

Reality hit shortly after I entered practice. One of my first patients was a man who had suffered a prolapse of his 5th lumbar disc; he complained during his second visit that he had passed a large and bloody stool. I could not remember any association between disc and such a clinical presentation, and did not know if this might have been associated with his disc as a sign of complication or if it might simply be an incidental finding. I did not know how to proceed, and I therefore referred him to an orthopedist. With time and more experience comes greater knowledge, which I sorely lacked in my early days. In part, this was due to my reliance on facts.

But education and clinical practice are, of course, so much more than facts. Clinical practice consists, in part, in knowing how to make appropriate clinical decisions and, in part, knowing how to find the answers to questions that arise in day-to-day practice. It is dynamic and it is for that reason that the shift toward problem-based learning (PBL) has arisen. Today, problem-based programs are occurring not only in clinical scientific education, but also in all aspects of academe. There is movement toward problem-based programs within chiropractic education. Both The National College of Chiropractic and Los Angeles College of Chiropractic have instituted problem-based programs: the Guided Discovery Curriculum at NCC and the Advantage program at LACC. Other chiropractic institutions, while not embracing full-blown PBL curricula, have added PBL classes within the framework of their overall curriculum. I know that the same is true in osteopathic education.

PBL brings with it new challenges. One is that textbooks play a different kind of role within PBL. Our standard textbooks offer lots of facts, and are indeed wonderful sources of information; however, they may not always be prepared in such a way that they would work best within a PBL program. That is why books such as Dr Spencer's are so very valuable. Problem-based medical education requires a new way of finding and using information; questions will arise in the natural course of working up a patient. The best texts, and the best courses, of a problem-based program bring together elements of both basic and clinical science in an integrative fashion. Dr Spencer's does this so very well. It asks students not only to concentrate on the diagnosis and treatment of the patient cases it discusses, but it also asks them to consider anatomical and physiological issues, as well as biomechanical and pharmacological issues. It fully integrates elements from all components of osteopathic education. It is case based. It is active, asking not only that the reader think about issues, but also that the reader should actually stop reading and go and *do* something. It requires active participation. This is so much more than the average text offers, and the material here can be applied to both osteopathic and chiropractic education, recognizing the many similarities our kindred professions share.

I am deeply honored to offer these words on behalf of Dr Spencer and his text. I know how very hard developing a book can be. This text is a significant addition to the manual therapy literature, one that I sincerely hope will be referred to again and again, until it is dog-eared from long overuse.

1997   D.J.L.

Preface

Have you ever sat in on a surgery with an experienced doctor or therapist? Did you marvel at the way they seemed to get to the heart of a problem with a few questions and a couple of examination steps? Did you go away thinking either 'that's easy' or 'how on earth did they do that'?

Well, let me tell you that behind that impression of ease is an enormous amount of knowledge and skill, which has usually been acquired by long hours of study and practice. The only way to gain the knowledge is to read the books, and the only way to gain the skill is by practice.

Why then, you may ask, produce yet another book to burden the poor student in his wearisome journey? Well, I think that this book is a little different from most of the others that I have seen. It is not a textbook of anything, and it is most certainly not a comprehensive textbook of anything. It is more a small collection of cases that I hope will help you to use your textbooks more effectively.

When I was a medical student, I found that the most useful way of remembering things was to relate them to actual patients I had seen on the wards. One of my first patients was a lady whose blood pressure I had to take, lying and standing, four times a day. I can still remember her face after nearly 25 years, and I can still remember the details about blood pressure control and treatment of hypertension that I associated with her! The next best thing to a real person is a case history designed to illustrate particular points. There are plenty of books of case histories, but these are usually tied to a particular subject, such as anatomy, physiology or neurology. They are very useful for studying these subjects, but unfortunately a patient does not present with an '-ology' but with a pain which you have to sort out.

This book is an attempt to get you to use your various textbooks, in the context of a person who might present to a practitioner, in order to study the case from several points of view. This is the so-called 'problem-based' approach, and it is becoming increasingly popular in training institutions. The cases are fictitious but based on real ones that I have seen in my practice, and I have made some attempt to make their stories memorable in some way. I have assumed that you are a private practitioner of a manual therapy (such as osteopathy, chiropractic or physiotherapy) and that you have access to special investigations such as blood tests and imaging. You will need a number of textbooks in various subjects such as:

— anatomy (including surface anatomy)
— biomechanics
— histology
— physiology
— pharmacology
— psychology
— sociology
— clinical examination
— differential diagnosis
— medicine
— orthopaedics
— research methods
— pathology
— radiology.

In addition to this, you will of course have the textbooks specific to your particular discipline. You will find a short list of textbooks that I have found useful at the end of the book, but I would emphasise that using a textbook is a very personal matter. Any book that you use should not be too simple, as there is sometimes a fair amount of detail required in the activities. At the end of each case there are one or two references to help you study the individual condition in a little more detail than is given in the average textbook.

Devon 1997   P.S.

Acknowledgements

This book would never have been started without the encouragement and support from my students and colleagues at the London School of Osteopathy. I have always felt that basing learning on a case study approach was helpful, and I have used this approach extensively in my lectures and tutorials. 'Write a book about it then', the students would taunt. So, not wanting to duck a challenge, here it is!

I also want to thank Dr Paul Treweeke from the department of radiology at North Devon District Hospital for collecting the radiological material, and Mr Dick Seddon of the department of biochemistry at the same hospital for photographing it. Paul said that collecting the radiographs was a 'nightmare', so I am definitely going to take him out to lunch to thank him (or perhaps give him something to make him sleep more peacefully).

Finally, the people who I want to thank most are my family, and especially my wife, who put up with me getting up at 5 a.m. each morning to work on this project, and also helped to type much of the material from my scrawl. 'When's it going to be finished, Dad?' are the words which will remain with me down the ages.

How to use this book

You will find a large number of activities to do. Some of them involve using everyday materials to illustrate a point. Hopefully they are fun to do, but do not get bogged down in the details of the activity and miss the point that it is trying to make. Other activities involve examining various parts of the body. You will need a partner for these activities, and I have assumed that you have a male partner. For most of the activities females are just as good for examination purposes. Many activities involve looking things up in your textbooks and these are indicated by the book icon. I have tried to link many of these to a 'doing' activity so that the reading becomes a little less tedious, but sometimes you just have to hit the books if you want to gain the required knowledge. Most of the activities are associated with a number of questions which I hope you will use to enhance your knowledge. They are of widely differing difficulty and take different times to complete. You might like to use them in a study group to make the learning into a social event as well as an educational task.

This is not primarily a textbook of differential diagnosis cases, but if you wish you can use it as such by just looking at the shaded text, which has the details of the history, physical examination and investigations, together with questions associated with these. They should help you to think about the clinical details of the case, and the detective work involved in forming a differential diagnosis. The discussion at the end of each chapter gives some idea of the approach that might be useful when faced with a patient who presents in a similar way to that of the case study. It is not meant to be a comprehensive discussion of all aspects of the case – this is, after all, what your textbooks are supposed to give you.

Since the book uses knowledge and skills from a wide variety of subjects, you may find that your course has not yet covered some of the material in the activities or questions. This is a difficult one to overcome, since your course has to start somewhere and build on knowledge and skills already gained. You may find that this book is useful to you at several stages of your course. Just pick out the activities and questions which are relevant to you at your particular stage, and keep the book handy for when you progress to a further level of competence. You may then view the case in a different light with your more advanced skills.

It has been difficult to decide which topics to include in each case. Some of the cases in this collection are quite complex, and could easily take a book in themselves. You might think that my choice is somewhat quirky. However, when you have gone through the whole book, you should find that you have covered quite a fair proportion of the topics of which a practitioner of manual therapy has to be aware.

One of the most important points about this book is that most of the cases are about patients who present to a manual therapist with history of musculoskeletal pain. It is essential to exclude non-musculoskeletal causes of the symptoms before assuming that the patient is suitable for whatever your particular brand of treatment happens to be. I hope that these cases will help to imprint this fact firmly in your mind. Do not forget, however, that most of the diseases described in this book are not all that common, so don't go around thinking that everyone suffers from the problems discussed here.

Finally, the objective in my writing this book has been to try to make your learning a bit more fun and a bit less 'dry'. The style is quite informal – I strongly feel that you don't have to write in formal language to make a point. Take as much time as you wish to do the activities, but do them thoroughly, and do think about the points that they are making. Good luck!

Introduction: the clinical method

Thomas Robinson, a 60-year-old farmer who smoked 30 cigarettes a day but had previously enjoyed very good health, went to see his doctor one busy morning surgery because he had been suffering from pains in the legs for the previous 2 months. The doctor asked Mr Robinson a number of questions about the pains, such as:

— Where exactly do you feel the pain?
— How long has the pain been there?
— Has the pain been getting better or worse over this time?
— What does the pain feel like?
— Is the pain there all the time?
— Does anything seem to make the pain worse or better?
— Do you have any other symptoms associated with the pain?
— Do the pains affect your work?
— Do you have any particular worries about the pains?

The doctor also asked some general questions about Mr Robinson's past medical history, his tobacco and alcohol intake, whether he was allergic to anything, and whether he was taking any regular medication. She also asked if there were any serious illnesses in his family.

Mr Robinson reported that he had not been feeling particularly well for about the previous 6 months, and that it was funny that the doctor should mention it but he had noticed having to get up two or three times during the night in order to pass urine. This had made him feel tired and thirsty when he got up in the mornings, and as a consequence his work at the farm was beginning to suffer.

When the doctor examined Mr Robinson, she first of all noted that he was moderately overweight. She then examined his legs; she first of all *inspected* the legs, looking for swelling, varicose veins, discolouration and any areas of irregularity in the skin. Next, she *felt* the legs, feeling for lumps or tenderness. She then felt in the groins, behind the knees and in the feet to determine whether there was normal pulsation of the arteries. She then performed a neurological examination on Mr Robinson's legs, testing for tone, power and coordination of the muscles, for impairment of sensation (using a piece of cotton wool, a pin and a tuning fork), and for the knee, ankle and plantar reflexes. She tested the hip, knee and ankle joints to determine whether there was any pain, restriction of mobility, or instability. She checked his blood pressure (it was high) and his heart. Finally she examined Mr Robinson's eyes with an ophthalmoscope.

The doctor then explained that she would like to test a small specimen of Mr Robinson's blood. She did this by using a special device which inserted a small lancet into a fingertip and produced a small blob of blood. This was picked up by a special stick with one end coated in a mixture of chemicals. The chemicals changed colour in response to the level of sugar in the blood. The test revealed that Mr Robinson's blood sugar level was higher than normal. The doctor explained that there were several possible reasons for Mr Robinson's leg pains, but that diabetes was quite likely. She took a sample of blood from a vein in his arm, and sent it to the laboratory. She told Mr Robinson to return in 1 week for the result.

A week later, Mr Robinson attended the doctor's surgery for the results. They showed that the level of glucose in the blood was 12 mmol/l, as opposed to a normal range of approximately 4–7 mmol/l. A diagnosis of diabetes mellitus was made. Since Mr Robinson was 60 years old, it seemed likely that he had the form of diabetes that did not require insulin injections. The doctor therefore started Mr Robinson on a weight reducing, low-fat diet which she advised him to try for 3 months. She also advised him to stop smoking, moderate his alcohol intake and continue to take regular exercise (his farm work was probably providing an adequate level of exercise). She took a further blood sample to check whether there was any infection or other factor which might have precipitated the onset of the diabetes, and sent Mr Robinson to the hospital for a chest X-ray and an electrocardiogram (ECG). All these investigations were normal.

Mr Robinson stuck rigidly to the doctor's advice, and when he returned to the surgery 3 months later he had lost 10 kg in weight, his blood pressure had returned to normal, and his blood glucose level was within the normal range.

The above description represents what might go on every day in a general practitioner's surgery. It illustrates the process known as the *clinical method*, which the practitioner uses to determine what (if anything) is wrong with a patient, and what to do about any abnormality. The basic steps are similar whether we are thinking about an 'orthodox' western general practitioner or a 'complementary' practitioner of acupuncture, osteopathy, etc.

The first step in the application of the clinical method is that the patient presents to the practitioner with one or more *symptoms*.

Questions for discussion

- Can you suggest some common symptoms?
- What knowledge is required at this stage?

At this point, it is important to realise that a symptom is not the same thing as a disease. There may be several possible diseases which give rise to a particular symptom. For example, swelling of the ankles may be caused by (among others) heart disease, kidney disease or liver disease as well as arthritis of the ankle joints. The clinical method is used by practitioners to help distinguish between these possibilities.

It is important to note that the doctor did not make her decision solely on the basis of the symptoms that Mr Robinson presented. There are other factors which a trained practitioner will need to know about which may not seem immediately relevant to the patient (such as the passing of excess quantities of urine in the case of Mr Robinson). This consideration leads us on to the second stage of the clinical method, namely *taking a history*. From the details given above, you will note that the case history consists of asking questions about many aspects of the patient's past and present health.

It is important when taking a history to develop good communication skills, for example:

— Be observant, open, honest and sensitive to the patient's needs
— Try to adapt to the patient and ensure that there is no misunderstanding over terminology
— Do not influence the patient into giving you the answer you hope for
— Never assume anything, always clarify a point
— Have a critical attitude to what the patient tells you.

History taking can be divided into:

— Presenting complaint
— History of present illness
— Past medical history
— Family history
— Personal and social history
— Review of systems.

Question for discussion

■ What do you think the significance of the questions about Mr Robinson's work and home life might be?

Having taken a history, the practitioner will have a mental list of possible diagnoses. This is the *differential diagnosis*. The next stage in the clinical method is to test these possible diagnoses to see if the range of possibilities can be narrowed down, ideally to a single disease.

Question for discussion

■ How did the doctor go about this in the consultation with Mr Robinson?

In the physical examination the doctor looked for *signs* of disease.

Questions for discussion

■ What is the difference between symptoms and signs?
■ What examination steps did the doctor perform on Mr Robinson?
■ Why did the doctor examine Mr Robinson's arterial pulses?
■ What skills are required at this stage?

The doctor also performed other examination steps to eliminate other causes of leg pain. In this case, the doctor was fairly sure that Mr Robinson had diabetes, and so she went on to test for *precipitating factors* and *complications* of diabetes. The signs revealed by the examination all pointed to a *diagnosis* of diabetes mellitus.

Questions for discussion

■ Having arrived at a probable diagnosis, what did the doctor do next?
■ What knowledge and skills are required now?

The process by which the final diagnosis is arrived at is a bit like detective work:

— The nature of the 'crime' is defined (e.g. murder, robbery)
— A hypothesis is set up regarding the motive
— A list of 'suspects' is drawn up
— Clues are gathered
— One by one the 'suspects' are eliminated or further questioned as to their involvement in the 'crime'.

In the clinical setting, the problem is defined as a set of symptoms, a differential diagnosis is formed and further information is gathered by taking the history, performing a physical examination and doing appropriate special investigations.

Question for discussion

■ What else, apart from making a diagnosis, did the doctor do?

When a diagnosis is made, the next questions to consider are:

— What is the likely outcome of the condition (*prognosis*)
— What *treatments* exist for the condition?

In the case of diabetes, there are a number of different approaches to treatment, varying from diet through tablets to insulin injections. Other aspects of *management* would include regular checks for complications, careful attention to foot hygiene and so on. If you read different textbooks, you might find that they have slightly different approaches to treatment and different criteria for applying each type of treatment.

Questions for discussion

■ Why might there be such variation in approaches to treatment?
■ What is 'evidence-based medicine'? Do you think that basing treatment on scientific evidence will help to improve the quality of treatments for particular conditions?
■ What knowledge and skills are required for this stage of the clinical method?

The prognosis can be quite difficult for the practitioner to determine. There are always occasions when a patient appears to have 'defied the doctors' by living longer than anticipated, and the opposite is true just as often. In other words, an assessment of prognosis is only an average of a large number of people with the condition.

Question for discussion

■ What factors can you think of that will influence the prognosis of a disease such as diabetes?

A final stage in the clinical method is the *follow-up*. This is usually a review of the progress of the patient at some later date after the diagnosis has been made and treatment instituted, although sometimes a diagnosis may not be made initially and the patient is followed up to determine how the clinical picture evolves, when a diagnosis may become more apparent. The effects of any treatment are also *evaluated* at this stage, and the doctor may wish to repeat some or all of the stages of the clinical method in order to check that the initial diagnosis was correct or to assess the progression of the symptoms, signs and special investigations.

Question for discussion

■ What difficulties can you see with the clinical method as described above?

I hope that you can see from this short introduction that there is an enormous amount of knowledge that you have to have before you can begin to apply your mind even to elucidating the cause of a particular set of symptoms, let alone to how to manage the patient who arrives on your doorstep wanting to be healed. Do not despair, however; if you hang your knowledge and skills on the cases that you meet, whether in this book or in real life, you will get there in the end.

Miss Tracey Gardener

Study objectives

After studying this case with its associated activities and questions, you should have a reasonable knowledge of the following areas:

1. The anatomy of the thoracic cage, with the surface anatomy of the most important structures
2. The movements of the thoracic cage during inspiration and expiration
3. The attachments, movements and nerve supply of the muscles of respiration
4. The attachments, movements and nerve supply of the diaphragm
5. The anatomy of the accessory muscles of respiration
6. The histology of the air passages
7. The physiology of air flow in tubes of varying diameter
8. The concept of the work of breathing, and how it changes with breathlessness
9. Simple lung function tests
10. Definition of asthma
11. Symptoms of asthma
12. Trigger factors for asthma
13. How to examine the chest
14. Physical signs in the chest with asthma
15. Examination of a normal chest X-ray
16. The chest X-ray in asthma
17. Complications of asthma
18. Drug treatment of asthma, including side-effects
19. Aims of manual therapy in the asthmatic patient.

Background

Miss Tracey Gardener, a 28-year-old primary school teacher, had suffered from asthma for most of her life. As a child, she had experienced moderately severe symptoms, consisting of cough, wheeze and shortness of breath, and had to have quite a lot of time off school. According to her story, she was 'always in Casualty with her chest'. However, the symptoms had abated somewhat since she had avoided dairy products in her diet. She was still quite wheezy and breathless after only moderate exertion, took her Ventolin and Becotide inhalers regularly, and if she developed a cold it usually progressed into a chest infection and she was 'laid up' for at least a week. On several occasions as a child, she had developed a more severe episode of breathlessness and wheezing, which had necessitated hospital admission and treatment with intravenous aminophylline and a short course of oral steroids.

It was after one of these chest infections that Miss Gardner came to see you, not about the asthma but on account of pain in the back of the upper thorax, extending across the tops of the shoulders and into the neck. This pain had been gradually increasing in severity for the previous 3 months.

Question for discussion

■ What questions would you ask Miss Gardener concerning her pain?

Miss Gardener told you that the pain was aching in character, and was made worse when she was breathless and easier when her breathing was better. The pain was also aggravated by rotating her head in either direction, but particularly to the right. There was no direct association between the pain and taking a deep breath. There was no extension of the pain down the arms, nor was there any headache. She was taking ibuprofen, an anti-inflammatory drug, which seemed to relieve the pain a little, but paradoxically seemed to make her breathing worse.

Questions for discussion

■ What do you think is the cause of Miss Gardener's neck pain?

■ Why do you think that the breathing might be worse with the anti-inflammatory drug?

Activity 1.1

▶ You will need your partner stripped to the waist for this activity. On your partner's chest identify the following landmarks:

— Sternum, with its component parts – what are they?

— Sternal angle, at the junction of the manubrium and body of the sternum

— 2nd rib, on either side of the sternal angle

— Spine of the scapula – with which thoracic spine is it level?

— Inferior angle of the scapula – with which thoracic spine is it level?

— 10th rib

— Clavicle

— Suprasternal notch

— Sternoclavicular joint

— Supraclavicular fossa

— Acromioclavicular joint

— Costal margin.

Activity 1.2

▶ Ask your partner to breathe quietly. Watch the expansion of the upper and lower parts of the chest. Measure this using a tape measure around the chest under the armpits and at the level of the xiphisternum. Note any abdominal movements that occur.

▶ Repeat this activity with your partner breathing slowly and deeply.

▶ Are there any differences in the abdominal movements between:

— The movements of the upper and lower parts of the chest?

— Quiet and deep breathing?

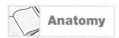

Anatomy

▶ Study the anatomy of the thoracic cage (see also Ch. 10 for
further information on the thoracic vertebrae). Concentrate,
for the moment, on the ribcage and sternum. Note the
following:

— The shape of the sternum, and its division into
manubrium, body and xiphoid process

— The articular surfaces on the superior surface of the
manubrium, on either side of the suprasternal notch, for
articulation with the clavicles

— How the 1st and part of the 2nd costal cartilages articulate
with the manubrium

— The sternal angle, where the body articulates with the
manubrium, and the notch for the articulation with part of
the 2nd costal cartilage

— The body also has notches for the articulation of the 3rd to
6th and part of the 7th costal cartilages

— The xiphoid process is quite variable in shape, but usually
has a facet for articulation with the 7th costal cartilage.

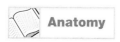

Anatomy

▶ Study the structure of the ribs and their connections to the
sternum and to the vertebral column. Note the following:

— The arch-like shape of the ribs, with its anterior end, shaft,
and posterior end

— The depression on the anterior end for the costal cartilage,
and the flattened shape of the shaft

— Note particularly the groove on the inferior surface of
the shaft, where the intercostal vessels and nerves
travel

— The head, neck and tubercle of the posterior end, where
the rib articulates with the vertebra.

▶ Study the general shape of the ribcage. Note that it is roughly
conical, broadening from above downwards, and flattened
from front to back.

Questions for discussion

■ What functions can you think of for the thoracic cage?

■ What is a 'cervical rib'? What symptoms might be experienced by a person with a cervical rib?

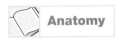 **Anatomy**

▶ Look at the anatomy of the joints between the ribs and the vertebrae, and the movements of the ribs at these joints. Note the following:

— The movement of the rib consists of a rotation whose axis passes through the costotransverse and the costovertebral joints

— The direction of this axis varies with the ribs, so that the lower ribs perform a 'bucket handle' motion while the upper ribs perform a 'pump handle' motion.

▶ Look at the anatomy of the joints between the ribs and vertebrae and work out why the movements of the upper ribs should differ from those of the lower ribs.

Questions for discussion

■ What is the effect of elevation of the ribcage on
  – the anteroposterior diameter of the lower thorax?
  – the transverse diameter of the lower thorax?
  – the anteroposterior diameter of the mid-thorax?
  – the transverse diameter of the mid-thorax?
  – the anteroposterior diameter of the upper thorax?
  – the transverse diameter of the upper thorax?

■ What is the effect of elevation of the ribcage on the position of the sternum?

Activity 1.3

▶ Ask your partner to run vigorously on the spot for a couple of minutes, until he is breathless. Note the following:

— Any differences in the rate and depth of breathing, and in the muscles used

— Note especially any contraction of the neck muscles, and the abdominal muscles.

▶ Wait until your partner has recovered his breath, and then ask him to try to breathe out forcefully against a closed mouth, so that no air comes out (a Valsalva manoeuvre). Ask him what happens to the abdominal muscles, neck muscles and diaphragm during this exercise. Feel the neck and abdominal muscles on your partner while he is performing the manoeuvre.

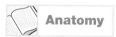 **Anatomy**

▶ Study the muscles that are involved in breathing, particularly the following muscles, their attachments, actions and blood and nerve supply:

— Levator costae

— Internal intercostal

— External intercostal

— Sternocostalis

— Diaphragm.

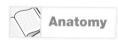 **Anatomy**

▶ Look at the diaphragm. Note the following:

— Its dome shape and its position, separating the thoracic and abdominal cavities

— The muscular fibres originating mainly from the lower vertebrae, ribs and costal cartilages, and converging to form a central tendon at the apex of the dome

— The main openings in the diaphragm to allow the passage of the aorta, inferior vena cava and oesophagus.

▶ Now study the effects of contraction of the diaphragm. Note that the central tendon is depressed, increasing the vertical diameter of the thorax in a similar way to the piston of a bicycle pump when it is pulled out.

Questions for discussion

■ What limits the depression of the central tendon?

■ Once the central tendon is fixed at the maximum level of depression, how does the diaphragm increase the transverse and anteroposterior diameters of the thorax?

- How does the diaphragm assist in such actions as
  - sneezing
  - coughing
  - laughing
  - crying
  - vomiting
  - defaecation
  - childbirth?
- How does the diaphragm act with the abdominal muscles during inspiration and expiration?

Activity 1.4

▶ If you can, ask someone who suffers from asthma what it feels like to be breathless during an attack. Ask if it is more difficult to breathe in or to breathe out.

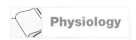 **Physiology**

▶ Study the movement of air in the airways during inspiration and expiration.

▶ Before you do this, you might like to make a model of the lungs and air passages. Cut the bottom off a plastic lemonade

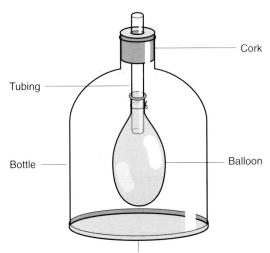

Cork

Tubing

Bottle

Balloon

Rubber stretched across cut end of bottle

Fig. 1.1 A model of the lungs and air passages can help you to study the movement of the air in the airways during inspiration and expiration.

bottle. Cut open a largish balloon so that it forms a flat sheet of rubber. Now stretch the balloon so that it covers the cut end of the bottle, and secure it with some thread. Get a cork with a hole in it (you should be able to get this from a shop which sells wine-making equipment), thread a piece of tubing through the hole and tie another (uncut) balloon onto the end of the tubing. Now fit the tubing into the neck of the bottle so that the balloon is inside the bottle (see Fig. 1.1).

▶ You now have a crude model of the chest. The cut balloon represents the diaphragm, and the balloon inside the bottle represents the lungs. Pull the 'diaphragm' downwards and watch what happens to the 'lungs'. Now release the diaphragm and watch the movement of the lungs.

Question for discussion

■ In what ways does this model differ from the situation in a real chest?

▶ Now put a restriction in the tube so that the diameter of its lumen is reduced to a very small value. Repeat the experiment, and see how long it takes for the air to enter and exit the lungs during the inspiratory and expiratory phases. If you push on the diaphragm, does the air exit the lungs more quickly?

Questions for discussion

■ Which muscles are responsible for normal quiet
  - inspiration
  - expiration?
■ What are the 'accessory muscles of respiration'?
■ What is the nerve supply of these muscles, including the spinal roots?
■ What happens to the diaphragm during:
  - quiet respiration
  - deep breathing?
■ What happens to the abdominal muscles when you are breathless?

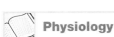 **Physiology**

▶ Study the measurement of respiratory movements by spirometry. Look at the following volumes:
  — Tidal volume
  — Inspiratory reserve volume
  — Expiratory reserve volume
  — Residual volume.

▶ Now look at the various combinations of these basic volumes into the lung capacities:
  — Vital capacity
  — Functional residual capacity
  — Total lung capacity.

Questions for discussion

■ You cannot measure the residual volume (or any of the capacities that include it) by spirometry. How could you measure the residual volume?

■ How might asthma affect these lung volumes?

Activity 1.5

▶ Move your head and neck to determine the range of motion that can be achieved. You should be able to flex your head forwards until the chin reaches the chest, and extend it backwards until the face is almost horizontal.

▶ Rotate the head in both directions – the chin should nearly reach the level of the shoulders – i.e. a 90° rotation in either direction.

▶ Tilt your head to one side so that the ear approaches the shoulder (without moving the shoulder). Now push your head directly forwards and backwards, without looking up or down. Finally, shrug your shoulders towards your ears.

▶ Repeat all of these movements, either on yourself or on your partner, while resisting them with your hand. As you attempt the movements, the muscles responsible for them will contract and you can see this as well as feel the contraction with your other hand. Contraction against resistance is, of course, the way in which muscle strength is tested in clinical practice.

Questions for discussion

- Which joints in the cervical spine are responsible for most of the rotation of the head?
- Which muscles are responsible for each of the movements you have demonstrated in Activities 1.1 to 1.5?
- Which nerves are you testing by performing each of the neck movements?
- Why do you think Miss Gardener has restricted head rotation?
- What might cause an asthmatic person to have a pain in the neck?

Activity 1.6

▶ Look at an anteroposterior X-ray of a normal chest in full inspiration. The best way to study any X-ray film is to be systematic about it. For a chest X-ray, it is probably best to examine the bony framework first, then look at the soft tissues around the thorax, then concentrate on the lung tissue and heart.

▶ Look at the scapulae first, then at the upper ends of the humerus and the shoulder joint. Next, look at the clavicles and finally the ribs, in pairs, from top to bottom. It is difficult to separate the spine and the sternum in this view because they are superimposed on each other and on the mediastinal structures.

▶ Study the soft tissues of the breast area, the supraclavicular area, the axillae and the sides of the ribcage. Check for the presence of female breasts, and for any asymmetry in the triangles of dark fat in the supraclavicular region.

▶ Look at the lung itself. The 'lung markings' (the branching linear shadows emanating from the hilum of the lung) are blood vessels. Look at the large vessels near the hilum; as shown here, the left hilar shadow is normally slightly higher than the right. Since you are looking at a normal film, there should be no abnormal patches of increased or decreased density on it indicating possible disease.

▶ Compare the level of the diaphragm on a normal film with that on a film from a person with asthma, such as Miss Gardener, whose lungs are hyperinflated. (It is also possible to observe the movements of the diaphragm in the living person using fluoroscopy.)

Questions for discussion

■ What is the 'diaphragmatic' shadow on a chest X-ray actually composed of?
■ What is the normal level of the diaphragm
  – in full inspiration
  – in full expiration?
■ What happens to the diaphragmatic levels when the chest is hyperinflated, as in asthma?
■ How would you expect the movements of the diaphragm and chest wall to differ from normal in an asthmatic patient?
■ What physical signs might you expect on examination of Miss Gardener's respiratory system?

Examination

Examination of Miss Gardener showed that she was quite a small lady with a barrel-shaped chest. Her head was protruded forwards on her shoulders, and she had an anxious expression on her face. She was not breathless at rest, but the respiratory pattern showed a markedly prolonged expiratory phase. There was no cyanosis or clubbing of the fingers. The trachea was not deviated from the central position. Chest expansion was symmetrical and within normal limits. The percussion note was judged to be hyperresonant, but there was no asymmetry. On auscultation of the chest there was reasonable air entry but there was a marked expiratory wheeze heard all over the chest.

Questions for discussion

■ Why do you think that the expiratory phase is prolonged in Miss Gardener?
■ What do you understand by the term 'cyanosis'?
■ How would you demonstrate cyanosis in a patient?
■ What is the difference between central and peripheral cyanosis?
■ Why might a person with asthma develop cyanosis?
■ What do you understand by the term 'clubbing' of the fingers?

- How would you demonstrate clubbing of the fingers in a patient?
- What causes can you think of for clubbing of the fingers?

Activity 1.7

▶ You will need two straws for this activity, one narrow and one wide. Try to breathe in and out through the wide one and then through the narrow one (pinch your nose to make sure you cannot cheat). You should find that it is much more difficult to breathe through the narrow straw. How long can you keep this up before you gasp for breath? Try to imagine what it is like to feel like this all of the time.

▶ While you are breathing through the straw, notice the effort required to get air in and out of the lungs, and how long it takes you to get each breath in and out. Note also the muscles that you use to force the air in and out.

▶ Write down the sensations that you feel as you are performing this activity. Do you feel 'breathless'?

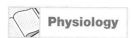 **Physiology**

▶ Study the mechanics of pulmonary ventilation. You have already looked at the change of shape of the thoracic cage during inspiration and expiration, and the muscles that cause these changes. Now look at the pressures involved in ventilation of the lungs. Note the following:

— The changes in pleural pressure and alveolar pressure during normal breathing

— The transpulmonary pressure, which is the difference between the pleural and alveolar pressures.

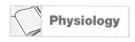 **Physiology**

▶ Look at a compliance diagram of the lungs. Have you ever seen people who blow up hot water bottles as a party trick? From our point of view, they perform a very useful function in that they demonstrate very graphically the principle of

compliance. Applied to the pulmonary system, this is the extent to which the lungs expand for a unit increase in transpulmonary pressure. The diagram you are looking at should show the pleural pressure plotted on the horizontal (x) axis and the lung volume change on the vertical (y) axis. You can see that the curves for inspiration and expiration are not the same.

▶ Place a small drop of tap water on a waxy surface. The water forms itself into a ball. This phenomenon is due to the surface tension of the molecules on the air/water interface. Now get some detergent, mix it with some more water and place a small drop of this on the surface near to the original drop. This time the height of the ball is less than previously because the detergent lessens the surface tension of the water molecules. If you try to float a razor blade on water, you will succeed only if the razor blade is dry and water does not get onto its upper surface. Think about why this should be so.

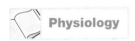 **Physiology**

▶ Study a compliance diagram of the lungs when they are filled with saline and compare this with the shape of the compliance diagram for the air-filled lung.

Questions for discussion

■ What is meant by 'airway resistance'?

■ Which airways provide most of the resistance in the lungs?

■ Why should the compliance of the saline-filled lung be less than that of the air-filled lung?

■ What is 'surfactant', and how does it work to lessen the compliance of the lung?

■ What is meant by the 'work' of breathing?

■ What proportion of this work is used to overcome airway resistance in normal breathing?

■ What happens to the work of breathing when you are breathless?

■ Which muscles were you using when you were trying to breathe through the straws, particularly the narrow one?

Activity 1.8

▶ Looking at the structure of the airways is important for an understanding of what goes on in asthma.

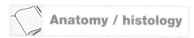 **Anatomy / histology**

▶ Look at the structure of the air passages. Note:
— The presence of smooth muscle and how this becomes more prominent further down the respiratory tract until the bronchioles have a continuous layer surrounding them
— How this muscle layer is arranged around the circumference of the bronchi and bronchioles
— The presence of hyaline cartilage in the larger airways, and how the presence of this diminishes in the smaller passages
— The presence of mucus-forming cells.

Activity 1.9

▶ Get a piece of string and form it into a loop (see Fig. 1.2).

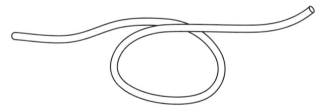

Fig. 1.2 To simulate constriction of the airways. Step 1.

▶ Now put a straw inside the loop and pull the ends of the string until it constricts the straw. Try breathing through the straw while it is constricted (Fig. 1.3).

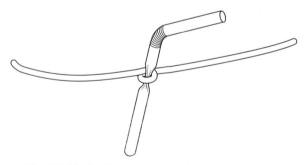

Fig. 1.3 To simulate constriction of the airways. Step 2.

▶ This is a bit like the sensation you get when the airways are constricted by contraction of the muscle fibres.

Activity 1.10

▶ Place a small piece of jelly or similar material into the straw. How easy is it to breathe through the straw now?

▶ This is a bit like the mucous layer of the air passages producing 'plugs' of mucus, again reducing the lumen of the airways, this time from the inside.

Activity 1.11

▶ Ask an asthmatic person if there is anything that seems to trigger an attack, for example exposure to dust, pollen or certain foods. Ask also if there is any asthma, hay fever or eczema in their family (blood relatives only). Allergies to various triggers appear to be inherited, but the manifestations may differ in different family members. Ask what a severe attack feels like – many sufferers say that they feel that they are going to die. Ask what medication they are on, and how they take it. Ask also if they are experiencing any adverse effects from the medication.

Questions for discussion

■ What is 'smooth' muscle? How does it differ from 'skeletal' and 'cardiac' muscle?

■ What factors cause smooth muscle to contract?

■ Miss Gardener had avoided dairy products and this had seemed to improve her breathing somewhat. Do you have any ideas about why this should be so?

■ What is an allergic response?

■ What are 'mast cells'? Where are they found? What is their role in the allergic response?

■ What is IgE? What happens when an allergen binds to an IgE molecule on the mast cell surface?

■ What is histamine? What is its role in the allergic response?

Activity 1.12

▶ Blow up a balloon, hold it by its neck and pull the neck so that you get a musical note as the air escapes. You can change the note by varying the tension with which you stretch the neck of the balloon. Experiment with this. Generally, you should find that the harder you pull, the higher is the pitch of the note, and the slower the balloon will deflate.

Question for discussion

■ How do you think the noises that are heard in Miss Gardener's chest are produced?

Activity 1.13

▶ This activity is designed to get you to start performing percussion. First of all, identify the middle finger of both hands. If you are right handed, lay the left hand flat on any surface (don't worry too much about what surface it is for the moment – you will soon be doing it on an actual chest). Now tap the middle finger of the left hand sharply, using the middle finger of the right hand. It is important to raise the right hand off the left hand almost as soon as the strike has been made. Use the tip (not the pad) of the right hand, and strike the left hand just proximal to the distal interphalangeal joint. The action should come mainly from the wrist, and the arm should hardly move at all. (If you are left handed, simply reverse the instructions.)

▶ Listen to the sound that is produced. If you have done it correctly, there should be a sharp sound rather than a prolonged muffle. Try the technique on several different surfaces and compare the sounds. Try it on yourself. Firstly, percuss over the lateral aspect of the hip joint, and then over the right hand side of the chest wall, a little below the clavicles. The sound produced when percussing the chest should sound more 'hollow' than when percussing over the hip area.

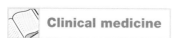 **Clinical medicine**

▶ Look at the examination of the respiratory system. You will see that it follows a logical order of inspection, palpation, percussion and auscultation. Generally speaking, percussion is often not well explained in the books, which is why I have gone into a little detail here, but the only way to become proficient in examination of the respiratory system, as in any other practical technique, is to practise, practise, and practise again, preferably under the initial guidance of an experienced supervisor.

Question for discussion

■ What tests would be the most useful for Miss Gardener's further management?

Miss Gardener's respiratory pattern shows a prolonged expiratory phase, suggesting that the airflow through the air passages is reduced. It is possible to quantify this by means of 'lung function tests'. There are many of these, and some are quite sophisticated and complex, but a relatively simple one that is used at home by many asthmatics is a peak expiratory flow meter (Fig. 1.4).

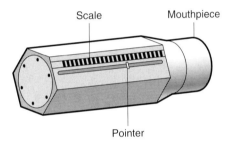

Fig. 1.4 A simple peak expiratory flow meter.

Activity 1.14

▶ If you have access to a peak expiratory flow meter, use it. Take a deep breath in, place your mouth over the mouthpiece and blow out as fast as you can. Record the reading. Repeat this twice more and take the highest of the three readings. You can then look up the normal value for yourself in a table of values.

▶ If you do not have a meter, take a deep breath in and force it out as quickly as you can. Think about the pattern of air flow as you are breathing out. A lot of air comes out initially, and then the amount of air being expired reduces considerably as you force the last bit out. Did the same thing happen with the balloon experiment in Activity 1.12?

Question for discussion

■ What factors could cause a reduction in peak expiratory flow rate?

A more complex test of lung function involves a spirometer (a device rather like a sophisticated paper bag), which can measure the volume of air inspired and expired and has a record of the time taken. A further refinement allows the flow rate to be calculated automatically from the recording.

Activity 1.15

▶ Look at the two graphs shown in Figure 1.5. They are spirometric recordings of the volume of air expired against time, for an expiration which is forced out as quickly as possible (a so-called 'forced expiration'). Graph **A** is normal and graph **B** is a recording from Miss Gardener.

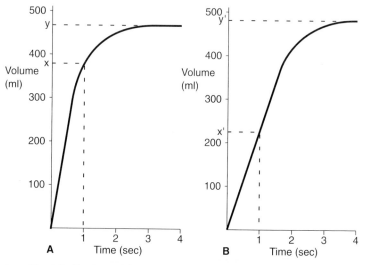

Fig. 1.5 Tracings of **A** normal, **B** abnormal spirometric recordings.

▶ First of all, look at the difference in the shape of the curves. Notice that in curve **A** the curve starts off steeply and then quickly flattens out, whereas curve **B** is much shallower and reaches the plateau more slowly. Think about what this tells you about Miss Gardener's ability to get the air out of her lungs.

▶ Look at recording **A**. The point marked x is known as the forced expiratory volume in 1 second (FEV_1), which tells you how much air you have breathed out in 1 second after starting a forced expiration. Point y is known as the forced vital capacity (FVC), which is the maximum volume you can breathe out after taking a deep breath and forcing the air out.

Points x^1 and y^1 are the corresponding points on recording **B**, Miss Gardener's record.

▶ Now calculate x/y and x^1/y^1. The answer you get is the FEV_1/FVC ratio, which is a very important measure of lung function.

In plain language, the FEV_1/FVC ratio is the proportion of the total breath that can be exhaled in the first second. In 'obstructive' lung disease like asthma, the airways are narrowed and resistance to air flow is increased, causing a prolonged expiratory phase and a low FEV_1; however, the total amount of lung ventilated is not reduced, and so the FVC remains normal, or even high if the lungs are hyperinflated. The FEV_1/FVC ratio is thus reduced. The normal value is above approximately 75%.

In 'restrictive' lung disease, such as emphysema, the calibre of the airways is not reduced but the amount of functioning lung is smaller than normal. This means that the FVC is reduced, but the fraction of the FVC that can be expired in the first second is normal. Thus the FEV_1/FVC ratio is normal.

Question for discussion

■ Why do you think there is such a difference between the two spirometric recordings in Figure 1.5?

Activity 1.16

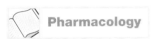
Pharmacology

▶ We know that Miss Gardener was using Ventolin and Becotide inhalers. Look up the action of salbutamol, which is commonly found as Ventolin in inhaler form. It acts in a similar way to adrenaline in the sympathetic nervous system, and its importance in asthmatics is that it dilates the bronchi. Think about what effect this would have on Miss Gardener's spirometric tracing (Fig. 1.5).

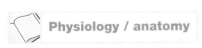
Physiology / anatomy

▶ Stimulation of the sympathetic nervous system produces effects other than dilatation of the bronchi. Look up these effects, then revise the details of the sympathetic and parasympathetic nerve supply to the lungs. Note the following:

— The lungs are supplied by nerves from the anterior and posterior pulmonary plexuses

— The input to these plexuses, especially from the vagus nerve and the sympathetic fibres from the 2nd to 5th thoracic ganglia on the sympathetic trunk.

Question for discussion

■ How far is it possible to predict the side-effects of the sympathomimetic drugs (drugs which mimic the effects of the sympathetic nervous system) from a knowledge of their actions on the organs of the body?

▶ Ventolin is called a bronchodilator, for obvious reasons. Think about other ways, apart from mimicking sympathetic nervous system activity, that bronchodilatation could be achieved.

Questions for discussion

■ What other bronchodilators can you find?

■ How do they act?

■ In what form are they administered?

■ What side-effects do they have, especially on the musculoskeletal system?

Bronchodilators such as Ventolin are usually given to relieve symptoms. Other drugs may be given to prevent attacks from occurring.

Disodium cromoglycate (Intal) may act by preventing the release of inflammatory mediators from mast cells. It is used regularly as a preventive measure, and has no direct bronchodilator action. It is administered as a 'spincap' which is inhaled.

Corticosteroids are powerful drugs which have an anti-inflammatory action. They also have some serious side-effects, especially when used orally over prolonged periods. However, the use of steroids by the inhaled route (e.g. Becotide) has dramatically reduced the incidence of these side-effects.

Questions for discussion

■ Which of the side-effects of corticosteroids are of particular relevance to manual therapists?

■ Do you think that any of these apply to Miss Gardener, given the clinical details that you have so far?

Activity 1.17

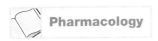 **Pharmacology**

▶ Miss Gardener found that taking ibuprofen for the ache in her neck produced a worsening of the breathing. Look up the action of ibuprofen. It belongs to a class of drugs known as non-steroidal anti-inflammatory drugs (NSAIDs). One of the unwanted effects of this type of drug is that it may worsen asthma in susceptible individuals. This class of drugs is widely used for general aches and pains, usually without a prescription from the doctor, so it is very important to be aware of the potential side-effects, particularly of gastric bleeding and exacerbation of asthma.

Drug treatment is of course only one aspect of the management of a patient with asthma. The main aims of treatment by a manual therapist are to:

— Reduce the work of breathing, or at least to ease symptoms due to the increased muscular effort required

— Ease removal of secretions

— Educate the patient regarding posture and breathing patterns.

Questions for discussion

■ How do you think Miss Gardener's job as a teacher affected her musculoskeletal problems?

■ What would you advise Miss Gardener regarding avoidance of triggering factors?

■ What views do you have about the role of the following in the development and maintenance of asthma:

   – air pollution
   – smoking
   – stress
   – exercise
   – poor housing
   – diet?

How would you go about investigating your ideas?

■ If Miss Gardener suddenly developed a pain in the right side of her chest, made worse by deep inspiration, what complication do you think would have developed? How would you confirm your suspicion? Is the condition dangerous? What would be the treatment of this condition?

■ What is 'status asthmaticus'? Is the condition dangerous? In general terms, how is the condition treated?

The American Thoracic Society defines asthma as 'a disease characterised by increased responsiveness of the bronchi to various stimuli, manifested by widespread narrowing of the airways that changes in severity either spontaneously or as a result of treatment'. It is essential for the diagnosis that the bronchoconstriction be at least partially reversible by inhaled bronchodilators. Many 'triggers' such as exercise, cold air, chest infections, drugs and industrial chemicals may start an attack. Asthma affects approximately 5% of children and 2% of adults in the UK – about 2000 people die each year from asthma, and some of these deaths may have been preventable.

The main feature of the asthmatic reaction is hypersensitivity of the bronchi. This leads to bronchoconstriction, inflammation and mucus production in response to appropriate triggers. This leads in turn to the clinical features of cough, wheeze and breathlessness, commonly worse at night. Physical signs on examination depend upon the severity of the condition. Chest wall deformity may occur in chronic asthmatics, especially if it has started in childhood. With a severe attack, the patient is distressed and vigorously contracts the accessory muscles of respiration. In such cases, air entry is greatly reduced because of the intense bronchospasm and the chest may be 'silent', i.e. no breath sounds can be heard. A severe attack that persists despite treatment is called 'status asthmaticus', and both this and chronic asthma may lead to respiratory and cardiac failure. In most cases, however, the breath sounds will be moderately reduced and there will be an expiratory wheeze resulting from the vibrations set up during the passage of air through the narrowed airways. Chronic mild breathlessness can lead to aching in the accessory muscles of respiration, which may then bring the patient to the attention of a manual therapist.

The main investigations are lung function tests, which show an obstructive pattern of respiratory disorder with a low FEV_1/FVC ratio, and the chest X-ray, which usually shows normal or hyperinflated lungs. Sometimes, plugs of mucus can cause collapse of a lung segment. Spontaneous pneumothorax, with a sudden exacerbation of breathlessness and acute chest pain that is much worse on inspiration, can be a complication in an acute attack.

FURTHER READING

Dodge R, Cline M G, Lebowitz M D, Burrows B 1994 Findings before the diagnosis of asthma in young adults. Journal of Allergy and Clinical Immunology 94: 831–835

Nielsen N H, Bronfort G, Bendix T, Madsen F, Weeke B 1995 Chronic asthma and chiropractic spinal manipulation: a randomised clinical trial. Clinical and Experimental Allergy 25: 80–88

Case 2
Miss Anne Harrison

Study objectives

After studying this case with its associated activities and questions, you should have a reasonable knowledge of the following areas:

1. Surface anatomy of the major structures in the lower leg, particularly those that may give rise to pain
2. Histology of skin
3. Anatomy of the tibia and fibula
4. Attachments and actions of the muscles in the lower leg
5. Testing of muscles, particularly in the leg
6. Functions of postural muscles
7. Nerves supplying the leg
8. Testing the neurological system in the leg
9. Histology of arteries and veins, and the differences between them
10. Arterial circulation in the leg
11. Palpating arterial pulses in the leg
12. Venous circulation in the leg
13. Blood flow in veins
14. Function of valves in the venous system
15. Anatomy of the microcirculation
16. Fluid flow in the microcirculation
17. The concept of osmotic pressure
18. The physiological mechanisms underlying oedema formation
19. Testing for pitting oedema
20. Causes of oedema
21. Differential diagnosis of leg pain
22. Blood clotting
23. Factors involved in thrombus formation
24. Pharmacology and side-effects of the contraceptive pill
25. Pharmacology and side-effects of anticoagulant drugs
26. Deep venous thrombosis in the leg
27. Contraindications to manual therapy in deep venous thrombosis.

Background

Miss Anne Harrison, a 24-year-old Parliamentary secretary, felt that life was very good to her. She had a good career with a very good salary and excellent prospects, a very comfortable flat in central London and a fast car. Her boyfriend and she both agreed that children were the last thing they wanted. Accordingly, she had decided to take the contraceptive pill at the age of 18, when she had commenced regular sexual intercourse. Her medical examination at the time she started taking the pill was entirely normal, and blood pressure checks since that time were also normal. The only problem that had troubled her recently was a mild pain in the right leg which had been present for about a week. Being the kind of person who did not want such a little thing to affect her life, she consulted you because you had successfully treated her boss for sciatica a couple of years previously, and he had been trouble-free since.

Questions for discussion

- What causes can you think of for the pain in the leg?
- What questions would you like to ask her about her symptoms?

Miss Harrison told you that the pain was confined to the right calf and seemed to be worse when she was walking, although it could occur at rest. There was no back pain, and there was no history of trauma. The leg felt slightly warm and tight, but the feeling was relieved to a certain extent by putting her feet up. There were no pins and needles or numbness, nor was there any weakness or incoordination of the leg. She had not noticed any discolouration of the leg. She smoked approximately 15 cigarettes per day and drank very little alcohol. There were no other symptoms.

When trying to decide on the cause of a person's pain, it is useful to make a start by considering the anatomy of the painful area.

Question for discussion

- What structures in the leg could give rise to pain?

Activity 2.1

▶ You will have to get your partner to bare his leg from the knee down for this activity. On your partner's leg, identify the following structures:
— Patella
— Head of fibula
— Tibial tubercle
— Medial malleolus
— Lateral malleolus
— Anterior border of tibial shaft
— Achilles tendon
— Gastrocnemius
— Soleus
— Tibialis anterior
— Tibialis posterior
— Flexor digitorum longus
— Flexor hallucis longus
— Extensor digitorum longus
— Extensor hallucis longus
— Flexor retinaculum
— Extensor retinaculum
— Common peroneal nerve winding round the fibular head.

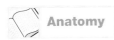 **Anatomy**

▶ Study the two long bones in the lower leg. Note the following:
— The tibia, which lies on the medial side of the leg, and is stout and strong
— The expanded upper end which articulates with the lower end of the femur and provides a good surface for the transmission of body weight
— The medial and lateral condyles where the menisci sit, and the intercondylar area where the cruciate ligaments are attached
— The shape of the shaft of the tibia, and, particularly, that the anterior border is subcutaneous for most of its length

— The lower end of the tibia with its medial malleolus, and the inferior surface for articulation with the talus bone of the foot.

▶ Look at the fibula, which is quite slender in comparison with the tibia. Note the following:

— It does not provide a surface for transmission of body weight

— The head of the upper end bears a facet for articulation with the lateral condyle of the tibia

— Note particularly that the lateral malleolus on the lower end of the fibula projects further down than the medial malleolus, and lies more posteriorly.

Activity 2.2

▶ Examine the skin of the leg. Is it hairy? (If you have a female partner, it might be diplomatic to avoid this question, but females do, of course, have a certain amount of hair on the leg, hence the popularity of ladies' shavers.)

▶ Pick up a fold of skin and gently squeeze it between your thumb and forefinger. Now let it go. Does the fold quickly disappear or does it take several seconds to go? As we get older the elasticity of the skin lessens, and so the fold of skin lasts for a much longer time. This loss of elasticity can also occur in dehydration.

 Anatomy / histology

▶ Look at a diagram of the skin. Note the division of the skin into the epidermis, dermis and subcutaneous tissue, and, in particular, the blood circulation, and the amount of subcutaneous tissue that is present. The epidermis varies greatly in thickness in different areas of the body, and the horny layer is greatly thickened in areas which are subjected to a lot of wear. Generally the dermis is made up of rather loose connective tissue, and so is able to hold quite a lot of fluid. Excess fluid in the interstitium is called oedema. The physiology of oedema production will be discussed later on in this case study, but for now you can learn how to test for oedema in the leg.

▶ With your partner lying supine, press your thumb firmly (but not too hard) into the centre of the dorsal aspect of the foot.

Press for about 20–30 seconds, and then take the hand away. Inspect the area that you have pressed. In a normal person there should be no impression left. If there is an impression, then the inference is that there is oedema. This sign is called 'pitting'. You can get some idea of what pitting oedema is like by pressing into a slightly over-ripe pear, but if you know anyone who has swollen ankles and will let you do it, you can feel the real thing.

Questions for discussion

- List at least six important causes of pitting oedema of the legs.
- Discuss the difference between the causes of unilateral and bilateral oedema.

Activity 2.3

▶ You will need a tape measure (not a steel one) and a marking pencil for this activity. With your partner lying supine, mark the most inferior point of the patella. Now measure 15 cm down the front of the leg and mark a point there. Take the tape measure and measure the circumference of the leg at this point, making sure that:

— The tape measure is not pulled tightly around the muscles of the leg

— The top edge of the tape is touching the mark.

▶ Compare the measurements for the right and left legs and determine whether there is a difference, and if so, how much it is. Repeat your measurements several times and determine how much variation there is. Get a few of your friends to repeat the measurements on your partner and ask them not to tell the others their results until everyone has made a measurement. You will be surprised at how much variation there is. If you have enough people you can construct a frequency histogram of the measurements.

Activity 2.4

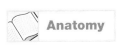 **Anatomy**

▶ Now you are going to look at the muscles of the leg. Study the attachments, actions, nerve supply and blood supply of the following muscles:

- Tibialis anterior
- Extensor hallucis longus
- Extensor digitorum longus
- Peroneus tertius
- Peroneus longus
- Peroneus brevis
- Gastrocnemius
- Soleus
- Plantaris
- Popliteus
- Flexor hallucis longus
- Flexor digitorum longus
- Tibialis posterior.

▶ As with any muscles, they are generally best seen when they are contracting against resistance. First observe the muscles for evidence of wasting. Now with your partner lying supine and fully relaxed, lift each knee in turn upwards about 15 cm. Repeat the manoeuvre with your partner tensing the leg muscles. Observe the movements of the foot. Is there any difference between the relaxed and tensed conditions?

▶ Ask your partner to perform the following movements while you try to stop the movements with your hands:
- Flex the knee
- Extend the knee
- Rotate the knee inwards
- Rotate the knee outwards
- Dorsiflex the foot
- Plantarflex the foot
- Invert the foot
- Evert the foot.

▶ Can you feel the belly of the individual muscles as your partner performs the movement? How strong is the movement?

There is an agreed nomenclature for the strength of muscle contraction:

0 – No contraction

1 – Flicker of movement
2 – Movement with gravity eliminated
3 – Movement against gravity
4 – Movement against gravity and resistance but weak
5 – Normal strength.

Questions for discussion

■ How can you eliminate gravity in each of the muscular movements?

■ What is the nerve root value of each of the movements?

Some of the muscles in the leg are 'postural' muscles, i.e. they help to maintain posture while standing. In the lower part of the leg, the gastrocnemius and soleus muscles are the most important ones to perform this function.

Activity 2.5

▶ With your partner standing still with feet placed approximately 15 cm apart, feel his leg muscles to determine whether they are relaxed or contracted.

▶ Repeat this with your partner standing on one leg (feel the muscles of both legs).

▶ Can you feel any difference between the leg on the ground and the leg off the ground?

▶ Some people like to stand with their weight predominantly on one leg, even though both feet are on the ground. Do this, and compare the muscle tensions in each leg.

▶ Get two sets of bathroom scales, and ask your partner to stand with one foot on each set and to adjust his posture so that he feels that his body weight is evenly distributed on each leg. Ask him to look directly forwards so that he cannot see the readings on the scales. Note the weight on each set of scales and determine how much difference there is.

▶ Now ask him to shift his weight onto one leg, and repeat the measurements. There should be a marked difference between the two sides.

Questions for discussion

■ What types of muscle fibre are present in muscles and how are postural muscles different in muscle fibre composition from muscles that have no postural function?

■ What long-term effects do you think that standing with your weight predominantly on one leg might have on the musculoskeletal system?

▶ Ask your partner to move the right heel up and down the left shin as quickly as possible. Repeat with the left heel and right shin. What do you think would happen with this manoeuvre if your partner had drunk a large quantity of alcohol?

▶ Now test your partner's knee, ankle and plantar reflexes. Have your partner lying supine on an examination couch. Put your left arm under his right knee and lift it a few centimetres from the couch.

▶ Hold the shaft of your reflex hammer near the end furthest from the head, and gently tap the knee just below the patella (you should be gentle but positive, and you should take the reflex hammer away from the knee as soon as it has struck the area). Note the response of the lower leg.

▶ Now bend your partner's knee a little further, and let the knee drop outwards so that the femur is abducted and the knee flexed. Grasp the foot with your left hand and hold it gently in dorsiflexion. Tap the Achilles tendon and note the response of the foot.

▶ Straighten your partner's leg. Now, run your thumb (or a car key) firmly up the lateral margin of your partner's foot, continuing across the inferior surface of the foot at the metatarsal heads. The toes should plantarflex.

Questions for discussion

■ Which nerve roots supply the ankle and knee reflexes?

■ What is the significance of an extensor plantar reflex (i.e. when the toes dorsiflex)?

The next few activities are concerned with the anatomy of the circulation in the leg, including the lymphatics.

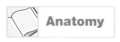

Activity 2.6

Anatomy

▶ To start with, study the arterial supply of the leg. The main feeding artery is the femoral artery.

▶ Follow the course of the femoral artery and its relations in the thigh. See how the femoral artery continues as the popliteal artery at the junction of the middle third with the lower third of the thigh. This then runs vertically downwards to the lower border of the popliteus muscle, where it divides into the anterior and posterior tibial arteries. The anterior tibial artery continues down the front of the leg where it continues along the tibial side of the dorsum of the foot as the dorsalis pedis artery.

▶ Identify and feel the pulsation of the femoral artery on your partner as it enters the thigh midway between the anterior superior iliac spine and the pubic symphysis.

▶ Identify and feel the pulsation of the popliteal artery. This is sometimes a little tricky, but you can usually feel it if your partner lies supine with the knee flexed to about 135°. Push up with both middle and ring fingers into the centre of the popliteal space, and move the fingers slightly laterally if you cannot feel it.

▶ Identify and feel the pulsation of the posterior tibial artery just posterior to the medial malleolus.

▶ Identify and feel the pulsation of the dorsalis pedis artery along a line from the mid-point between the two malleoli to the proximal end of the 1st metatarsal space.

Question for discussion

■ Where would be the best places to press on the arterial systems of the leg if a patient sustained a cut to one of the arteries?

Activity 2.7

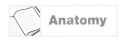 **Anatomy**

▶ Study the venous drainage of the leg. Notice in particular that there is a system of superficial veins and a parallel system of the deep veins, with communicating veins connecting the two systems.

▶ With your partner standing, identify the venous arch on the dorsum of the foot. Follow it to the short saphenous vein behind the lateral malleolus and the long saphenous vein in front of the medial malleolus.

You are now going to do some simple experiments on the veins which were first performed in the second quarter of the 17th century by the physician William Harvey (1578–1657). Before Harvey, it was thought that the blood ebbed and flowed from the heart. Harvey was the first to demonstrate that the blood moves 'in a circle' from arteries to veins. He could not see the capillaries which we now know connect the arterial and venous systems, and so he postulated a system of tiny 'pores' through which the blood flowed. Nevertheless, the demonstration of the circulation of the blood was a major advance in our knowledge of the body.

Activity 2.8

▶ With your partner supine, either wrap a blood pressure cuff around his calf and inflate it to about 60 mmHg, or else tie a piece of cloth reasonably tightly about the calf. In either case, the veins of the leg should become more prominent.

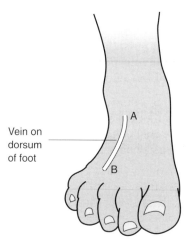

Vein on dorsum of foot

A

B

Fig. 2.1 Use a length of vein on the dorsum of the foot, such as the one shown here, to demonstrate the circulation of the blood.

Question for discussion

■ Why should the veins become more prominent when you constrict the calf?

▶ Next identify a good-sized vein on the dorsum of the foot. Identify any branching points and choose a length of vein free of such branches (see A–B in Fig. 2.1).

▶ Now put your left finger at A and the forefinger of the right hand next to it. Whilst still pressing on the vein, run your right forefinger up to point B. Note that the vein empties. Now take away the finger at A from the vein. Finally, take away the finger at B from the vein.

You should find that when you take the finger at A away, the vein fills up quickly, whereas taking the finger at B away results in the vein staying empty.

Questions for discussion

- What does this experiment tell you about
  - the direction of blood flow in the veins
  - the presence of valves in the veins?

Activity 2.9

▶ Have your partner lie supine. Raise his legs to about 45°. What happens to the veins? Can you still feel the arterial pulsation in the foot?

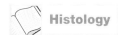 **Histology**

▶ Look at the differences between the structure of the walls of the arteries and that of the veins. This will help you to explain why the veins collapse when your partner's leg is raised while you can still palpate the arterial pulsations.

▶ If you know anyone with varicose veins, ask them to show you the dilated and tortuous superficial venous system. Such people may tell you that their ankles swell if they have been standing for long periods. You may also notice areas of brownish discolouration around the medial malleolus; this is called varicose eczema, which is a feature of poor oxygenation of the tissues. This may progress to ulceration if the condition is severe.

Questions for discussion

- Why should the ankles swell in a patient with varicose veins?
- Why is the oxygenation of the tissues of the leg reduced in a patient with ankle oedema?
- On which parts of the examination would you concentrate in Miss Harrison?

Activity 2.10

 Clinical examination

▶ You have already performed much of the medical examination of the leg in the previous activities. Now is the time to review these. In order to bring the various aspects of the leg together into a smooth examination, you will need to examine:

— The arterial circulation
— The venous circulation
— The motor system
— The sensory system
— The joints
— The bones.

 Medicine

▶ You will also need to think about examining the spine for referred pain, and the abdomen for evidence of blockage to the veins. Which features in the history might distinguish the pain arising from different structures?

Examination

Examination of Miss Harrison's legs showed that there was a mild degree of swelling of the right calf, but no discolouration. The right calf was slightly warmer than the left, and there was a tender area posteriorly in the middle of the gastrocnemius area. Right foot dorsiflexion increased the calf pain. Straight leg raising was 90° on both sides, reflexes in the lower limbs were normal, and there was no sensory or motor deficit. Peripheral pulses in the legs were all present and full. The leg joints were normal, as was the lumbar spine.

Questions for discussion

■ What do you think the diagnosis is now?
■ Which investigations might confirm your diagnosis?

- What would be your management of Miss Harrison?
- As a manual therapist, what treatment would you avoid?

Activity 2.11

▶ For this activity you will need a balloon and a length (about 60 cm) of clear plastic tubing (such as is used in winemaking). Tie the neck of the balloon around one end of the tubing. Next fill the balloon to the neck with water (it might be advisable to do this activity over a sink or bath). Figure 2.2 shows the general arrangement of the experiment.

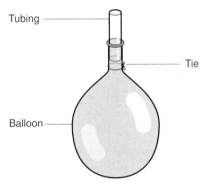

Tubing

Tie

Balloon

Fig. 2.2   A simple experiment using a balloon and a length of clear plastic tubing, arranged as shown here, demonstrates the manner in which the venous valves lessen the hydrostatic pressure in the veins and capillaries of the leg.

▶ Now, squeeze the balloon. As expected, the water rises in the tube. When you let go of the balloon, the fluid falls in the tube and the balloon expands with the water.

▶ Squeeze the balloon again. Now, before you let go of the balloon, squeeze the tubing so that the water above the tubing cannot fall through the constrictions. What happens when you let go of the balloon now? You should find that the water above the constriction stays above it, and that the balloon does not expand as much when you release the pressure on it.

The constriction in the tubing is acting as a valve and lessens the hydrostatic pressure in the balloon. In the same way, venous valves lessen the hydrostatic pressure in the veins and capillaries of the leg. In a person with varicose veins, these valves become incompetent and so the hydrostatic pressure in the capillaries rises.

Activity 2.12

▶ You will need the tubing that you used for Activity 2.10. Pierce the tubing near to one end with 10 to 20 small holes. Hold the tubing in a V-shape and fill it up. Put a cork or bung into the end of the tubing with the holes in it. Now lift up the other end of the tube and see how the water flows out of the holes that you have made (see Fig. 2.3).

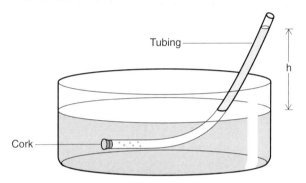

Fig. 2.3 The height (h) of the free end of the tube, and the size of the holes in the tube influence the rate at which the water flows out of the tube.

▶ Experiment with this by varying the amount by which you lift the free end of the tube, and then by making a few bigger holes near the small ones. You should find that the higher the free end is above the end with the holes, and the larger are the holes, the faster the water flows out of the holes.

▶ Draw two graphs of flow rate versus the height of the water column (h in Fig. 2.3) above the stoppered end of the tube, the first for the situation where you just have small holes and the second for when the larger holes are added.

Question for discussion

■ What does this experiment tell you about the relationship between flow rate out of the tube and

– pressure
– leakiness of the tube.

This experiment demonstrated two of the factors involved in the formation of oedema, namely:

— Raised venous hydrostatic pressure

— Increased permeability (leakiness) of the capillaries.

In fact, anyone might develop oedema of the legs if they stood for too long, if it were not for the fact that the leg muscles contract and 'pump' the blood up the veins towards the heart. This is called the 'muscle pump'. The venous valves also need to be competent in order to lessen the hydrostatic pressure in the veins of the lower leg.

A third factor which might cause oedema is a blockage of the lymphatic system. This system runs in parallel with the blood system, and its function as far as fluid dynamics is concerned is to soak up excess fluid and protein in the interstitium. Imagine that in Activity 2.12 there was a pipe leading out of the water tank at a certain level. Once the water level rose above the level of the pipe, any excess would be drained away (see Fig. 2.4). If the drainage pipe were blocked the fluid level would rise. If the level of water in the tank represents fluid in the interstitial space, then blocking the outflow of water would cause oedema.

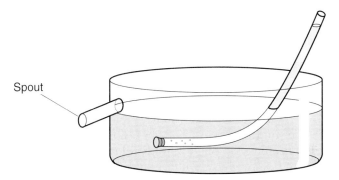

Spout

Fig. 2.4 The lymphatic system helps to drain away excess fluid and protein. A blockage can cause oedema, just as a blockage in this spout would cause the water level in the tank to rise.

The lymphatic system can only be directly seen in the normal living person at the lymph nodes (glands). If there is infection in the superficial tissues, you may see a red line along the lymphatic vessels leading to the lymph nodes. In the leg you may be able to palpate some lymph nodes in the groin.

Activity 2.13

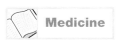

Medicine

▶ Find out the causes of enlarged lymph nodes.

Activity 2.14

▶ This activity demonstrates a fourth factor which may cause oedema, decreased blood osmotic pressure. You will need a large potato, water, some sugar and a bowl. (You will also need a few days!) Peel the potato and cut a core at one end (Fig. 2.5). Put it in the bowl. It is a good idea to slice off the bottom of the potato so that it is stable. Now pour some tap water into the bowl. Next, make a strong solution of sugar in water (use hot water to dissolve the sugar and then let it cool). Put some sugar solution about halfway up the well in the potato, and leave it for a couple of days.

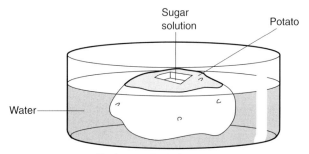

Fig. 2.5 An experiment to demonstrate osmosis. Decreased blood osmotic pressure is another factor which can cause oedema.

▶ You should find that the level of fluid in the potato well has risen, and it may even have flowed over the top of the potato back into the bowl.

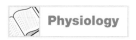 **Physiology**

▶ Study the phenomenon of osmosis as applied to fluid flow in the microcirculation.

Questions for discussion

■ What is osmotic pressure?

■ Which molecules are responsible for most of the osmotic pressure in blood?

■ Where are these molecules synthesised?

■ Can you think of any diseases in which there is a reduction in the osmotic pressure of the blood?

Now is the time to review the subject of fluid exchange in the microcirculation, and the causes and development of oedema.

▶ Review Activities 2.10 to 2.13.

 Anatomy / physiology / medicine

▶ Find out:
— The anatomy of the microcirculation (arterioles, capillaries, venules, lymphatic capillaries, interstitium)
— The dynamics of fluid exchange (Starling's hypothesis of capillary exchange, which should not be confused with Starling's law of the heart, just two of the enormous contributions made to physiology by Ernest H. Starling (1866–1927))
— The mechanisms underlying the formation of oedema
— The main causes of oedema.

Question for discussion

■ Which of the mechanisms of oedema formation do you think apply to Miss Harrison?

Activity 2.15

▶ Think about the last time you had a minor cut. The bleeding might seem to go on for ever, but eventually it stops and a clot forms, leading to a scab, which then slowly heals leaving either no trace of the injury or a small scar.

 Physiology / pathology

▶ Study the events that occur in response to a small cut. You should find that there are several processes:
— Local vasoconstriction
— Platelet aggregation
— Clotting of the blood
— Resolution of the clot
— Healing of the tissue.
▶ Note the following:
— Initial vasoconstriction causes a slowing of the local blood

flow, and allows the platelets to adhere to the damaged endothelium

— The platelets then release chemicals which activate a series of chemical reactions resulting in the formation of fibrin

— There is a cascade of chemical reactions involving the activation of the various clotting factors and an amplification of the amount of chemical formed at each step

— The action of fibrin in forming a network of cross-linked fibres stabilising the platelet plug

— The action of plasmin and other enzymes which are capable of breaking down the fibrin network.

Questions for discussion

■ What is the role of calcium in the coagulation process?

■ Where are most of the clotting factors synthesised?

■ What factors stop the blood from clotting inside the blood vessels?

■ What factors promote blood clotting inside blood vessels?

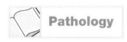 **Pathology**

▶ Study Virchow's triad, which is the name given to the factors predisposing to thrombosis. The triad may be summarised as:

— Damage to the vessel wall

— Reduction in blood flow

— Increase in blood clottability.

Questions for discussion

■ What are the clinical risk factors for thrombosis?

■ Which, if any, of these apply to Miss Harrison?

■ What is the difference between a thrombosis and an embolus?

■ What are the possible outcomes of thrombus formation?

Activity 2.16

▶ Miss Harrison smoked and was taking the contraceptive pill. Find someone who is taking the contraceptive pill. Ask her:

— What she knows about its side-effects

— How she is being monitored by her doctor
— Whether she smokes.

Questions for discussion

■ What are the side-effects of the contraceptive pill?

■ What other factors may interact with contraceptive pill use to increase the risk of thrombosis?

■ What evidence can you find regarding the relationship between contraceptive pill use and the incidence of cancer of the uterus, ovary, cervix and breast?

 Pathology / pharmacology

▶ Find out how contraceptive pill use can alter a number of laboratory investigations, e.g.:

— Prothrombin level
— Platelet aggregability
— Blood glucose levels
— Levels of clotting factors.

Question for discussion

■ If you suspected that Miss Harrison had a deep venous thrombosis (DVT) what investigations would be useful?

▶ Look at Figure 2.6. It is a photograph of a venogram. This is an X-ray of the leg which is taken with radio-opaque dye injected into one of the veins in the foot. The veins are outlined by the dye, and any defects in the lumen of the vessel (filling defects) may be seen.

Questions for discussion

■ Can you see any filling defect in the photograph?

■ What is the major complication of a deep venous thrombosis?

■ What manual techniques should be avoided in Miss Harrison?

■ What do you think the medical management of Miss Harrison should be?

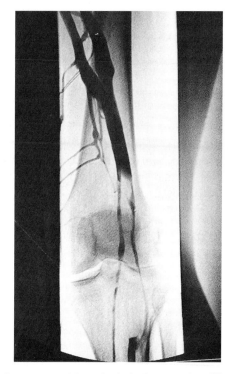

Fig. 2.6 A venogram of the veins in the leg may show filling defects.

Activity 2.17

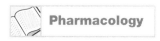 **Pharmacology**

▶ Study the different types of anticoagulants. You should find that there are:

— Inhibitors of platelet functions, e.g. aspirin

— Inhibitors of the coagulation cascade, e.g. heparin, warfarin

— Activators of fibrinolysis, e.g. streptokinase, tissue-plasminogen activator (TPA).

Questions for discussion

■ Which of the above agents may be given orally, and which have to be given by injection?

■ What is the major complication of these agents?

- What additional complications does aspirin give rise to?
- From the point of view of the manual therapist, what precautions would need to be taken with a patient on anticoagulants?
- Is there any interaction between aspirin and warfarin?

Diagnosis

Miss Harrison was referred immediately to her general practitioner, who arranged urgent hospital admission. A venogram showed a filling defect, and a diagnosis of deep venous thrombosis was made. She was anticoagulated, initially with heparin 48 000 u/24 h and then with warfarin sufficient to maintain the prothrombin ratio between 2.5 and 3.0. She was taken off the contraceptive pill and strongly advised to stop smoking.

Questions for discussion

- What is meant by the 'prothrombin ratio'?
- What psychological effects do you think Miss Harrison might suffer from:
  - having the thrombosis
  - having to stop the contraceptive pill
  - having to stop smoking?

Discussion

Pain in the leg is mostly due to neurological, vascular or musculoskeletal causes. It is therefore necessary to examine all these systems in a case of leg pain. In the case of Miss Harrison, there is no previous history of peripheral vascular disease, she is young and the peripheral pulses are all present, making intermittent claudication (due to blockage of the arterial supply to the leg) highly unlikely. The pain is exacerbated by walking, but also occurs at rest and so there is no consistent mechanical factor in pain generation. Swelling of the leg and local tenderness are not generally features of sciatica. There is no history of trauma but a musculoskeletal condition such as a spontaneous muscle tear or a ruptured Baker's cyst must still be considered. However, in a young lady taking the contraceptive pill and with a history such as that of Miss Harrison, the most likely cause is venous thrombosis.

Normally, thrombus formation is prevented by three factors:

— A smooth endothelial lining in the vessel wall
— Streamlined blood flow, preventing platelet contact with the endothelium
— The fibrinolytic system, which lyses any thrombi formed spontaneously.

There are thus three types of situation in which thrombus formation is more likely: abnormalities of the vessel, low blood flow, and hypercoagulability of the blood. Major risk factors for venous thromboembolism include immobility, dehydration, varicose veins, leg or pelvic trauma, surgery, pregnancy, heart failure, use of the contraceptive pill, cancer and obesity.

Deep venous thromboembolism (DVT) is a particularly insidious problem because the first clinical indication of its presence may be a massive pulmonary embolism. Pain is the most common symptom, being typically aching in character and aggravated by walking. The most reliable sign is swelling of the affected extremity, due to venous pooling and oedema due to the high venous pressure. Homan's sign (increased tenderness on foot dorsiflexion) is not a very reliable sign of DVT, and is now regarded as dangerous to perform in that it may dislodge a thrombus.

Clearly, the major risk with a person with a DVT is the subsequent development of a pulmonary embolism, which produces an area of lung which is ventilated but under-perfused, thus increasing the physiological dead space. Massive pulmonary embolism can cause sudden death. However, more subtle symptoms such as a worsening of a pre-existing cardiorespiratory condition may be associated with multiple small emboli. From the point of view of the manual therapist, *any* form of massage or soft tissue work on the affected leg is absolutely contraindicated, as is any articulation to the surrounding joints. Treatment is with anticoagulant drugs, and use of the contraceptive pill must be stopped. Urgent referral to the general practitioner, or even to hospital, is required.

FURTHER READING

Beyth R J, Cohen A M, Landefeld C S 1995 Long-term outcomes of deep-vein thrombosis. Archives of Internal Medicine 22: 1031–1037

Pasi K J, Perry D J, Lee C A 1995 Thromboembolism and the combined oral contraceptive pill. [letter] Lancet 345: 1437

After studying this case with its associated activities and questions, you should have a reasonable knowledge of the following areas:

1. Surface anatomy of structures in the hip and pelvic areas
2. Anatomy of the femur
3. Anatomy of hip joint and its movements
4. Testing of hip joint movements
5. Attachments, actions, blood supply and nerve supply of muscles acting on the hip joint
6. Blood supply of buttock, hip and upper leg
7. Nerve supply of buttock and hip areas
8. Histology of arterioles
9. Inter-relationships between pressure, flow and resistance in the circulation
10. Physiology of muscle blood flow control at rest and during exercise
11. Factors influencing the supply of, and demand for, oxygen in skeletal muscle
12. Energy supply for skeletal muscle contraction
13. Pathology of atherosclerosis
14. Pathophysiology of blood flow restriction in peripheral vascular disease
15. Major sites of peripheral vascular disease
16. Causes of peripheral vascular disease
17. Symptoms and physical signs of peripheral vascular disease
18. Contrast radiology in peripheral vascular disease.

Background

Mr Gordon Lennox, a 62-year-old Scottish bank manager, had taken early retirement, and was a keen golfer. He was looking forward to playing a major part in his local team's satisfactory progress in the forthcoming tournament. In preparation for this, he embarked on an exercise programme, which included a brisk 3-mile walk every day. On the first day, after walking about half a mile, he began to experience some mild discomfort in his right calf and more troubling pain in his right hip. After resting for a few moments, the pain subsided and he was able to continue. However, the pain recurred after about 10 minutes' walking and he found that if he continued to walk he began to limp. He had never had any leg trouble in the past, and when he returned home he was quite despondent. His wife, who had suffered from osteoarthritis of the hip for a long time, assured him that his symptoms were similar to hers, and that a course of homoeopathic medicines would help him as it had helped her. Accordingly, he visited his local homoeopath who prescribed a number of remedies to him over a period of 3 months, mostly with little improvement in his condition. He had already had to cry off from the golf tournament and was feeling pretty miserable. Eventually, he decided that seeing an osteopath might help his problem and so he came to see you with the above story.

Questions for discussion

■ Do you think Mr Lennox has a hip problem?

■ What other possibilities can you think of for the symptoms?

■ What further questions would you ask Mr Lennox?

Mr Lennox told you that the pain was aching in character, but that after walking for a few minutes it became progressively more like cramp in the calf, and became so intense that he had to stop. After a minute or so of rest, however, the pain subsided and he was able to carry on. Climbing stairs also brought on the pain in the calf. Mr Lennox did not complain of any other symptoms at all. He had no pains in any other joints, nor was the right leg swollen, hot or discoloured. He had no pain in the low back or the abdomen, and he regarded his general health as very good. 'If it wasn't for this stupid leg, I'd be as fit as a fiddle', was how he put it to you, and he was proud of the fact that despite having smoked more than 30 cigarettes a day for over 40 years, he had no chest problems at all and never became breathless.

Question for discussion

■ On which aspects of the physical examination would you concentrate in Mr Lennox?

We will start this case by reviewing the structures that can cause pain in the hip area. It is important for the patient to define exactly where the pain is, since patients may say that they have 'hip' pain if the pain is located anywhere from the groin to the buttocks.

Activity 3.1

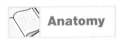 **Anatomy**

▶ You will need your partner to strip to his underpants for this activity. Identify the following structures on your partner, using your textbook as necessary:

— Iliac crest

— Anterior superior iliac spine

— Pubic tubercle

— Pubic symphysis

— Greater trochanter of femur

— Posterior superior iliac spine

— Spinous process of 4th lumbar vertebra

— Spinous process of 5th lumbar vertebra

— Coccyx

— Ischial tuberosity

— Sacrum

— Inguinal ligament.

Activity 3.2

▶ Ask your partner to stand upright with his knees and feet together. Note the obliquity of the femoral shafts, which are separated at the upper end by the width of the pelvis and are approximated at the knees in this position. Does your partner have 'bow-legs' or 'knock-knees'? Note that the base for supporting the weight of the body is quite narrow.

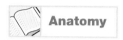 **Anatomy**

▶ Study the bones of the pelvis and the femur. There is more information on the hip bone itself in Chapter 14, but for this case you should concentrate on the upper end of the femur and its articulation with the hip bone.

▶ Look at the femur, which is the longest and strongest bone in the body. Note:

— The general shape of the femur, with its shaft and upper and lower ends

— The upper end of the femur, which consists of the head, neck, and greater and lesser trochanters

— That the head of the femur projects from the medial side of the shaft

— The shape of the head of the femur; it forms more than half a sphere, and is directed medially, upwards and slightly anteriorly (if you look at an articulated skeleton, you will see that the head of the femur is encircled by the acetabulum of the hip bone, up to its largest diameter)

— The fovea at the centre of the acetabular surface, which gives attachment to the ligament of the head of the femur

— The close relationship of the femoral artery and the psoas major muscle to the anterior surface of the head of the femur

— The angle that the neck makes with the shaft (this angle gradually diminishes from birth until adulthood).

▶ Look at pictures of skeletons of children and adults to confirm the diminishing angle noted above. The angle is also greater in the female, due to the greater width of the pelvis.

▶ Look at the greater and lesser trochanters, which serve for the attachments of muscles acting on the hip joint. Note the intertrochanteric line anteriorly, which marks the lateral limit of the capsular ligament of the hip joint. Posteriorly lies the intertrochanteric crest.

Questions for discussion

- What differences in structure and function can you think of between the shoulder and hip girdles?
- Which muscles have an attachment to
    - the greater trochanter
    - the lesser trochanter?
- How is the lower limb adapted for the upright stance?
- How is the lower limb adapted for walking?

Activity 3.3

▶ Ask your partner to lie supine on a couch or on the floor. Now bring his knee up towards his chest with his knee flexed. You should find that the knee can be brought up to almost touch the chest. The thigh then makes an angle of at least 120° to the spine. However, not all of this is hip flexion. If you place one hand under your partner's lumbar spine while you are flexing the hip, you will find that the spine appears to press down on your hand as the hip flexion reaches approximately 90°. This is because the pelvis is rotating around a transverse axis.

▶ With your partner's legs fully extended, grasp one ankle and pull the leg outwards into abduction. Note the angle that the leg makes with the sagittal plane of the body. Now pull the leg to the opposite side into adduction, and again note the angle that the leg makes with the sagittal plane. It is important to make sure that the pelvis does not move while you are performing these movements, otherwise your measurements will be erroneous.

▶ Flex your partner's right leg so that the thigh is vertical. Raise the lower leg so that it is horizontal (i.e. both hip and knee joints are flexed to 90°). Hold the knee with your left hand and grasp the right ankle with your right hand. Now rotate the hip joint by pulling the ankle to your partner's right and then to his left, being careful to keep the thigh vertical.

▶ Think about the last two movements. Which of them is internal rotation of the hip, and which external rotation?

▶ Finally, have your partner lie prone on the couch. Grasp one
of your partner's knees and raise it so that the hip is extended
as far as it will comfortably go. Measure the angle between
thigh and couch.

Questions for discussion

■ Which movements of the hip joint are involved in
   - doing the 'splits'
   - sitting with your legs crossed
   - squatting
   - sitting in the 'lotus' position
   - walking?

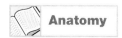

Activity 3.4

Anatomy

▶ Study the structure and movements of the hip joint. It is a ball-
and-socket joint, formed by the head of the femur rotating in
the acetabulum of the hip bone. The convexity of the femoral
head matches the concavity of the acetabulum. Compare this
with the situation in the shoulder joint. The acetabulum is
deepened considerably by the acetabular labrum, a ring of
fibrocartilage which encircles the rim of the bony fossa.

▶ Look at the capsular ligament of the hip, which is roughly
cylindrical in shape, and extends from the rim of the
acetabulum to the upper end of the femur. Note the following:
— The exact attachments of the lateral end of the capsular
   ligament, and the folds of capsule which allow some
   increase in hip abduction
— The direction of the fibres in the capsule.

Questions for discussion

■ How does the capsular ligament of the hip affect the range of
movement at the hip joint?

▶ Look at the following ligaments around the hip joint:
— Iliofemoral
— Pubofemoral
— Ischiofemoral.

▶ Examine the attachments of these ligaments and how they are coiled around the femoral neck.

Questions for discussion

■ Which movements of the hip joint
  − tighten the ligaments
  − loosen the ligaments?

■ How do you think the ligaments of the hip help a person to maintain the erect posture?

■ Why can the position of hip flexion be regarded as a 'position of instability'?

In the next activity you are going to investigate the muscles of the hip region by asking your partner to perform some movements which you resist. For each of these movements, observe the contraction of the muscles, and feel them tightening if you can.

Activity 3.5

▶ Have your partner lie supine on an examination couch. Stand at his right side. Place your right hand on his right knee and ask him to raise the knee against your resistance. Now place your right hand under your partner's right knee, raise it a couple of centimetres and ask him to press his knee downwards.

▶ Place your hands on the lateral aspect of both knees and ask your partner to separate the knees against your resistance. Then ask your partner to separate his knees by about 20 cm. Place your hands on the medial aspect of both knees and ask him to push his knees together while you resist.

▶ Finally, raise your partner's thigh so that it is vertical and the lower leg is horizontal. Place your left hand on your partner's right knee to stabilise it, and grasp his right ankle with your right hand. Then ask him to rotate his right foot to the right and then to the left, while you resist each movement in turn.

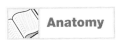 **Anatomy**

▶ Study the muscles that produce movement at the hip joint. For each of the following groups of muscles, note the attachments, actions, blood supply and nerve supply:

— Hip flexors
  - psoas
  - iliacus
  - sartorius
  - rectus femoris
— Hip extensors
  - gluteus maximus
  - biceps femoris
  - semitendinosus
  - semimembranosus
— Hip abductors
  - gluteus medius
  - gluteus minimus
  - tensor fasciae latae
— Hip adductors
  - adductor magnus
  - adductor longus
  - adductor brevis
  - gracilis
— External rotators of the hip
  - piriformis
  - obturator internus
  - obturator externus
  - gemelli
— Internal rotators of the hip
  - tensor fasciae latae
  - gluteus minimus
  - gluteus medius.

It is very important to note that most of these muscles have more than one action, and it is more useful to think of the muscles involved in a particular movement than of the individual actions of a particular muscle. Note the root values of the individual movements of the joint, and also the location and referral pattern of the trigger points of individual muscles.

Questions for discussion

■ Which muscles stabilise the pelvis when you stand on one leg
  – with the hip extended
  – with the pelvis tilted posteriorly
  – with the pelvis in anteroposterior equilibrium
  – with the pelvis tilted anteriorly?

Activity 3.6

▶ Ask your partner to walk slowly around the room and observe him. Note that, with each step, the leg on the ground is fully extended. This means that the joint capsule, ligaments, fasciae and flexor muscles are stretched repeatedly. Regular walking is thus a good exercise to prevent contracture of the hip flexor muscles, with its resultant adverse effect on gait.

▶ Ask your partner to try walking with the leg on the ground slightly flexed at the hip; he will tell you that it is much more difficult to do.

▶ Observe the rotation and tilt of the pelvis, and the flexion of the knees during walking.

 Anatomy / physiology / biomechanics

▶ Study the phases and determinants of gait (see also Ch. 11 for more activities on walking).

Question for discussion

■ What do you think would happen to the gait if one hip were arthritic and had a degree of fixed flexion, adduction and external rotation?

Activity 3.7

▶ Ask your partner to stand on one leg. Feel the contraction of the abductor muscles of the hip. You will see that the pelvis tilts upwards on the non-weight-bearing side.

It can be roughly estimated that the hip has a pressure of three times the body weight imposed on it when the opposite leg is off the ground (see Fig. 3.1). This happens because the distance of the centre of gravity of the body from the fulcrum at the centre of the hip joint is twice the distance between the fulcrum and the point of attachment of the balancing force of the hip abductors.

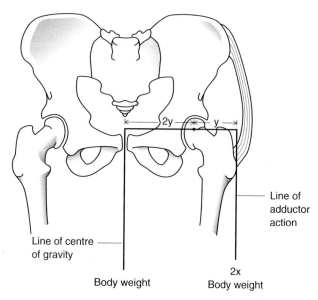

Fig. 3.1 To illustrate the increased pressure on the hip when the opposite foot is lifted from the ground.

▶ To illustrate this further, get two weights, one of 100 g and the other of 200 g, and tie a length of thread around each of them so that they can be hung up. Get a 30 cm ruler and balance it on a fulcrum (such as your partner's finger) to represent the centre of the hip joint. Now hang one weight on each end of the ruler. Adjust the ruler so that it is back in balance. Measure the distances from the fulcrum to the point where the weight hangs on each side; you should find that the distance to the heavier weight, representing the force of the hip abductors, is half the distance to the lighter weight, which represents the body weight (see Fig. 3.2). The total weight (not including the ruler) is 300 g, which is three times that of the body.

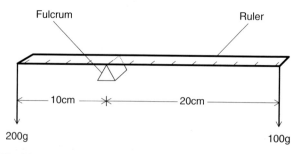

Fig. 3.2 The fulcrum represents the hip joint, and the lighter weight the body weight.

This force on the hip occurs every time you stand on one leg and during the stance phase of walking (see Ch. 11). This is why it is so important to advise overweight individuals with arthritic hips to lose weight.

Questions for discussion

■ What effect do you think that a walking stick might have on the pressure on the hip while walking?

■ Should you hold the walking stick on the affected side or the non-affected side? Give your reasons.

Activity 3.8

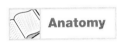 **Anatomy**

▶ Study the blood vessels supplying the buttock and hip areas. Firstly, follow the course of the common iliac artery as it branches from the aorta and then itself divides into internal and external iliac arteries. Note the external iliac artery becoming the femoral artery at the mid point of the inguinal ligament, after it gives off the inferior epigastric artery.

▶ Palpate the femoral artery on yourself or your partner.

▶ Study the course of the internal iliac artery as it runs just in front of the sacroiliac joint and gives rise to vessels which supply the pelvic organs, the gluteal and perineal regions, the iliopsoas muscle and the muscles of the posterior abdominal wall.

There is more information on the internal iliac artery in Chapter 14. For the moment, concentrate on the anatomy of the external iliac artery and the upper part of the femoral artery.

▶ Note the following:

— The close relationship of the external iliac artery to the psoas muscle, the ureter and the intestines as it travels downwards and laterally from its origin to the point where it becomes the femoral artery

— That the inferior epigastric and deep circumflex iliac arteries are the only branches of the external iliac

— The close relationship of the femoral artery to the hip

adductor muscles, the femoral nerve and vein and the hip joint

— The course of the following major branches of the femoral artery in the upper part of the thigh:
  - superficial epigastric
  - superficial circumflex iliac
  - superficial external pudendal
  - deep external pudendal.

▶ Study the profunda femoris artery arising from the lateral aspect of the femoral artery. This provides the main blood supply to the adductor, extensor and hamstring muscles. It also is involved in a number of important anastomoses, particularly with branches of the external and internal iliac arteries.

▶ Look at the branches of the profunda femoris artery, particularly the following:
  — Lateral circumflex artery
  — Medial circumflex artery
  — Perforating arteries (usually three)
  — Muscular branches.

▶ Look at the important anastomoses on the back of the thigh, which extend from the gluteal region to the popliteal region, as follows:
  — Gluteal arteries with the medial femoral circumflex artery
  — Femoral circumflex arteries with the first perforating artery
  — Perforating arteries with each other
  — Perforating arteries with muscular branches of the popliteal artery.

▶ Finally, study the blood supply of the hip joint. It comes from branches of the gluteal arteries running along the ligament of the head of the femur, anastomosing with branches of the medial and lateral femoral circumflex arteries at the trochanteric anastomosis.

Question for discussion

■ If a person sustains a fracture to the neck of the femur, what might happen to blood supply to the femoral head, and what might be the consequences?

Activity 3.9

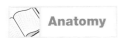 **Anatomy**

▶ Study the nerves of the buttock and hip areas. Again, there are more activities and information on this topic in Chapter 14, to which you are strongly advised to refer. For this case, consider the structures that can be the origin of pain in this area, and note the nerve supply of each of the following:
— Capsule of hip joint
— Joint synovium
— Ligaments of hip joint
— Muscles surrounding hip joint
— Periosteum
— Skin
— Subcutaneous tissue.

▶ Look at the following nerves which supply the hip joint and its surrounding structures:
— Femoral nerve
— Obturator nerve
— Inferior gluteal nerve
— Superior gluteal nerve
— Sciatic nerve
— Branches of the lumbar plexus
— Branches of the sacral plexus.

▶ Note that:
— The nerves supplying the short muscles of the hip also supply sensory fibres to the capsule of the hip joint
— Note particularly the relationship of the sciatic nerve to the piriformis muscle. In over 10% of people, some or all of the sciatic nerve passes through the piriformis muscle rather than just anterior to it. Spasm or contracture of the piriformis may then give rise to buttock pain radiating down the leg, which may be confused with similar symptoms arising from a prolapsed intervertebral disc or a stenosis of the lateral intervertebral canal.

Question for discussion

■ To which areas of skin can pain originating in the hip joint be referred? What is the anatomical reason for this?

Examination

When you examined Mr Lennox, you found that indeed he appeared to be surprisingly fit. His blood pressure was normal and his chest remarkably clear for a life-long smoker. Examination of the hip, which had actually never been performed previously, was entirely normal. There was no pelvic abnormality, and only a mild degree of restriction at the level of L5 on the right-hand side. The only medical abnormality that you found was that all the pulses in his right leg were absent, whereas the pulses on the left leg were palpable.

Questions for discussion

■ Have you managed to work out what the main problem is?

■ What investigations might be helpful in Mr Lennox's case?

■ Why should Mr Lennox's pain get worse with walking?

■ Which blood vessels are involved in the pathological process?

■ What can be done for Mr Lennox's arterial problem?

The next activity is a little different from the usual ones, but I hope that it will help you to grasp the principles of supply and demand. Have you ever gone into a shop for a particular item, only to be told that they don't stock it, with the annoying explanation that 'there's no demand for it'?

Activity 3.10

▶ Next time you visit a supermarket or corner store, think about their stock-control system. You might even ask the manager or shopkeeper about it.

The key to success with stock control is to monitor:

— How fast the particular item is selling

— How much reserve stock the shop has

— The time delay between ordering the item and delivery to the shop.

It is also very important to be able to predict how fast the item will sell in the future. It would be inefficient for the store manager to buy in, for example, a huge load of winter coats when winter was just ending just because they had sold well in the winter. It would be even worse if the item had a limited shelf life, such as fresh meat or vegetables.

Questions for discussion

■ In this system, what factors might cause a shortage of the item on the shelves?

■ What factors might cause a build-up of the item on the shelves?

A similar process happens at home. You need household items such as food and cleaning materials (demand). You estimate how much of these you need in the coming days or weeks and buy in the goods according to the principles outlined above. When you have used the goods, you dispose of the waste products. Sometimes, you decide not to go shopping and use up some of your stock of food, etc. If you were locked in your house with the windows and doors barred, and the toilet facilities were not working, you would soon find that there was a build-up of waste materials in the house (which is why refuse collectors can create so much disturbance if they go on strike).

Similar principles can be applied to the body's requirements for energy. The tissues are active, and in order to maintain this activity they have a certain requirement for oxygen and nutrients. This has to be supplied by the blood circulation, which also carries away the waste products of metabolism to the parts of the body where they are eliminated. If there is a blockage to the circulation, there will be a shortage of supply of nutrients and a failure to eliminate the waste products of metabolism.

In the next few activities, you will consider in a little more detail the question of supply and demand for oxygen in skeletal muscle.

Activity 3.11

▶ Perform some vigorous activity such as running on the spot until you are breathless and sweating. Note how the following have changed immediately after this exercise:

— Respiratory rate
— Depth of breathing
— Pulse rate
— Force of contraction of the heart.

Clearly, you will not be able to measure all of these accurately, but you can get an idea of the changes by listening to your body. You should have noted that all of the above factors increased during the exercise, and gradually returned to normal within a few minutes of stopping (depending on how fit you are!). Exercise is a good way of increasing the body's demand for oxygen and nutrients, and the body usually responds by increasing the intake of oxygen from the air (via the increased depth and rate of ventilation) and increasing its distribution to the tissues (via the increased rate and force of pumping of the heart).

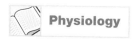 **Physiology**

▶ Find out what is meant by the terms 'cardiac output' and 'oxygen consumption', and find out how they change with vigorous exercise. You will also see that most of the increased cardiac output during exercise goes to skeletal muscle.

Question for discussion

■ How does the body increase local oxygen supply if you are only exercising a relatively small part of the body (for example, lifting a weight with your right arm)?

Activity 3.12

▶ For this activity, you will need to assemble the following objects: a length of clear, flexible plastic tubing; a funnel, attached to one end of the tubing; a jubilee clip to fit around the tubing; a ruler; and a watch with a second hand. A means of holding the funnel at various heights would be advantageous, but if you don't have anything suitable, ask your partner to hold the funnel steady while you perform the measurements. You will also need a jug of water and a beaker or other receptacle to catch the water when it flows out of the tube.

▶ Fill the tubing with water via the funnel. Stop the water from exiting the tubing by compressing the far end with your finger and thumb. Hold the funnel end of the tube vertical and ask your partner to mark two lines on the tube approximately 20 cm apart (see Fig. 3.3).

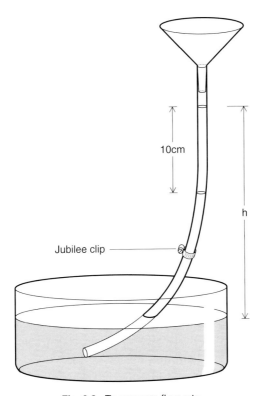

10cm

h

Jubilee clip

Fig. 3.3 To measure flow rate.

▶ Now unblock the free end of the tube and watch the water flow out into a receptacle. You can measure the flow rate in at least two ways:

— By measuring the time it takes for the water level to fall between the two marks on the tube

— By collecting the water coming out of the tube in, say, 10 seconds and weighing it.

Questions for discussion

■ Which of these two methods gives the actual flow rate and which gives a relative indication of flow rate?

■ How could you determine the diameter of the tubing (assuming that it is circular and uniform along the length of the tube) using the two methods combined?

▶ Repeat the procedure with the funnel at different heights (h) above the free end, and plot a graph of flow rate (on the y-axis) against height of funnel above the free end (on the x-axis). You should find that you get a straight line, the slope of which is the resistance to flow.

▶ Now tighten the jubilee clip so that the tubing is constricted but not completely closed off. Repeat the above measurements and determine the resistance to flow when the tube is constricted.

Activity 3.13

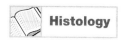 **Histology**

▶ Study the structure of arterioles. Note that, in common with all blood vessels except capillaries, they possess three coats:
— Tunica intima (inner layer)
— Tunica media (middle layer)
— Tunica adventitia (outer layer).

▶ Look at the layer of smooth muscle arranged concentrically around the arterioles. This can contract and relax, and has a similar effect to that of tightening and loosening the jubilee clip in the experiment you have just performed. Note particularly the nerve supply to the arterioles, which comes mainly from the autonomic system.

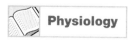 **Physiology**

▶ Study the factors that affect the local blood flow in a tissue.

One of the most important functions of the circulation is to allow individual tissues to control the local blood flow in proportion to their need for:

— A supply of oxygen and other nutrients (such as glucose, fatty acids and amino acids)

— Removal of waste products (such as carbon dioxide and hydrogen ions)

— Transport of specific substances (such as hormones or antibodies)

— Maintenance of a constant chemical environment in the tissue

— Special requirements of individual tissues (such as heat loss from the skin, excretion from the kidneys).

The blood flow through resting muscle tissue is quite low, yet during strenuous exercise it can increase by anything up to 20 times the resting level. In heavy exercise such as running, around 80% of the total cardiac output of the body can go to the working muscles. Clearly, tissue metabolism is a major factor in determining the diameter of the arterioles in the working muscles, and thus the resistance to blood flow through the tissue.

Question for discussion

■ Do you think that a vasodilator substance, produced during increased tissue metabolism, is responsible for the observed increase in blood flow, or do you think that local oxygen lack is the main factor in the vasodilatation? Give reasons for your answer.

Whatever the cause of the vasodilatation, it is clear that the greater is the exercise, the more the arterioles dilate. This is just what the muscle requires, since more blood, and therefore more oxygen and nutrients, can be delivered.

Activity 3.14

▶ A little mathematics may help to fix in your mind the scale of the increase in muscle blood flow and oxygen requirement during exercise. For the purposes of your calculation, you will need the following quantities:

- — Cardiac output (CO) in l min^{-1}
- — Percentage of CO going to muscles
- — Oxygen content of arterial blood in ml l^{-1}
- — Oxygen content of venous blood in ml l^{-1}.
▶ Assume that the following values occur at rest:
  - — 5 l min^{-1}
  - — 20%
  - — 200 ml l^{-1}
  - — 150 ml l^{-1}.
▶ Assume that the following values occur during strenuous exercise:
  - — 25 l min^{-1}
  - — 80%
  - — 200 ml l^{-1}
  - — 100 ml l^{-1}.
▶ First, calculate the amount of blood flowing through the muscles per minute. This is clearly the cardiac output multiplied by the percentage of the cardiac output going to the muscles. Next, determine the amount of oxygen extracted from each litre of blood as it passes through the muscles. This is the arterial oxygen concentration minus the venous oxygen concentration. The oxygen consumption is then calculated as the product of the two quantities you have just worked out.

You should have calculated that at rest, the muscle blood flow is 1 l min^{-1} and during exercise it rises to 20 l min^{-1}. This represents an increase of a factor of 20. The oxygen consumption goes up even more, from 50 ml min^{-1} to 2000 ml min^{-1}. The enormous increase in oxygen delivery to the working muscles occurs via three mechanisms:

- — An increase in cardiac output
- — A greater percentage of the cardiac output goes to the muscles
- — More oxygen is extracted from the blood as it passes through the muscles.

There are other factors, apart from arteriolar dilatation, which affect the flow of a fluid such as blood in a tubular vessel. One of these is the viscosity of the fluid.

Activity 3.15

▶ You will need a narrow straw, a wide straw, some water and some thick milk-shake for this activity (choose a flavour you like). Suck up some water through the narrow straw. It should be fairly easy.

▶ Repeat the exercise with the wide straw; you may not notice much difference, but it may be a little easier.

▶ Now suck up some thick milk-shake through the wide straw; you should find some resistance to the flow of fluid in the straw.

▶ Repeat this with the narrow straw. What happens to the straw? Can you suck up any milk-shake through the narrow straw?

▶ Cut the straws so that they are only about 5 cm long, and try to suck up the milk-shake again. Is there any difference in the resistance to flow?

Activity 3.16

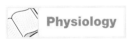 **Physiology**

▶ A little more mathematics, I'm afraid. Study the factors which affect the flow of liquids in tubes. You may come across Poiseuille's law, which is often expressed in the formula:

$$F = \pi r^4/8\eta l$$

where
F = flow rate
π = ratio of circumference of a circle to its diameter
r = radius of the tube
η = viscosity of the fluid flowing through the tube
l = length of the tube.

If you are not familiar with mathematical equations, do not despair. They are merely a shorthand way of expressing what can be said in words. This equation tells us that if the radius of the tube increases then the flow rate increases, while if the length of the tube or the viscosity of the fluid increases, the flow rate decreases (you have already discovered this in Activities 3.12 and 3.13). The important thing to note is that the equation also tells us that the flow rate increases as the fourth power of the increase in radius. This means that if the radius doubles, the flow rate increases by a factor of 16 (2 × 2 × 2 × 2). In the body, the length of the blood vessels and the viscosity of the blood are both fairly constant, and so the main determinant of peripheral resistance to blood flow is the calibre of the blood vessels, particularly the arterioles.

Now you are going to study some aspects of the demand for oxygen and nutrients in muscle. You have already seen (Activity 3.14) that the amount of oxygen taken up by the muscles during vigorous exercise can increase to many times the resting level.

Activity 3.17

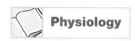 **Physiology**

▶ Study the chemical aspects of muscle contraction.

There are further activities on the mechanics of muscle contraction in Chapter 12. In that chapter, the emphasis is on cardiac muscle, but there are many similarities between the contraction of cardiac and skeletal muscle. For this activity, it is sufficient to be aware that adenosine triphosphate (ATP) provides the energy for the muscle filaments to slide along each other and produce contraction.

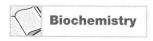 **Biochemistry**

▶ You can study how food and oxygen react to form ATP, but this would require a whole book in itself. Suffice it to state here that there is not enough ATP stored in the muscles to sustain maximal muscle power for more than a few seconds, and so it has to be formed continually during exercise. Note the following:

— There are several mechanisms for the production of ATP:
- creatine phosphate
- glycogen
- aerobic system
— The aerobic mechanism is the only one that can sustain exercise for an indefinite period, and so this system is used mostly for long-distance and endurance exercise

— For sprinting and other short-term vigorous activities, the other systems are used but they build up a 'debt' of oxygen which must be 'repaid' when the activity is finished.

Questions for discussion

■ How many molecules of ATP are produced from one molecule of glucose when it is metabolised:
  – anaerobically
  – aerobically?
■ What mechanism of ATP generation do you think will be used by the body when you go for a long walk?
■ Which waste products are produced by:
  – anaerobic metabolism
  – aerobic metabolism?
■ How is the oxygen debt paid off?

Now that you have studied some of the determinants of oxygen supply and demand in muscles, it is time to take a look at what happens when the supply cannot keep pace with the demand.

Activity 3.18

▶ You will need a blood pressure cuff or tourniquet for this activity. Inflate the cuff to above arterial pressure on your partner's arm, or tie the tourniquet tightly so that the radial pulse is abolished (NB: you should not under any circumstances keep the cuff inflated or the tourniquet tied for more than 10 minutes, even if your partner feels no pain).

▶ Ask your partner to exercise both hands simultaneously by squeezing a soft object, such as a tennis ball, in the palm of the hand. Your partner should do this quite vigorously.

▶ Ask him to note whether there is any difference in sensation in the two hands. There should be a gradual development of pain in the hand of the arm where the artery is occluded. Can you explain why?

When a muscle requires more oxygen than can be supplied, it is said to be ischaemic. From the previous activities, you know that the most likely cause of ischaemia is narrowing of the blood vessels, causing increased vascular resistance to blood flow. In the western world, the most common cause of this is atherosclerosis.

Activity 3.19

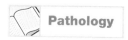 **Pathology**

▶ Study the appearances of atheromatous plaques. Other lesions, such as fatty streaks and intimal cushion lesions, are thought to be precursor lesions for the plaques. Note the structure of the plaque, with its fibrous cap and soft yellowish centre comprising lipid, foam cells and cellular debris.

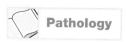 **Pathology**

▶ There is uncertainty as to how atheroma is produced. Assess for yourself the relative claims of the 'reaction to injury' hypothesis and the 'monoclonal' hypothesis. For the purposes of a manual therapist, it is not necessary to debate this particular issue in great detail; it is sufficient to know that atherosclerosis causes narrowing of the blood vessels and thus can give rise to ischaemic pain.

Questions for discussion

■ Which are the most common sites for development of atheroma?

■ What are the major risk factors for the development of atheroma?

■ How common is peripheral vascular disease?

■ Do you think that Mr Lennox's symptoms fit in with peripheral vascular disease?

Activity 3.20

▶ Finally, look at the photograph of the X-ray investigation shown in Figure 3.4. The investigation is called a digital subtraction angiogram.

▶ Note the narrowing of the common iliac artery. This confirms the diagnosis of buttock claudication due to stenosis of the common iliac artery.

Questions for discussion

■ How is a digital subtraction angiogram performed?

■ What complications of this investigation can you think of?

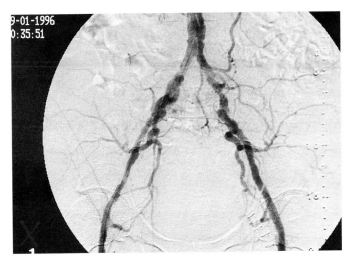

Fig. 3.4 A digital subtraction angiogram showing narrowing of the common iliac artery.

Discussion

As you probably realised fairly early on in the course of this history, Mr Lennox's problem had nothing to do with his hip. Claudication in the buttock is often confused with pain arising in the musculoskeletal system, but there are some clear differentiating points. The pain of osteoarthritis is very often worse on waking, before any activity has been undertaken, and is often relieved by gentle exercise. The pain of claudication is made worse by exercise, and there is often a 'claudication distance' that the patient can walk before the onset of pain. The pain is then relieved by rest, and then the patient can walk on for a similar distance.

The next question to decide is whether the claudication is due to a vascular or a neurological cause. Claudication of the cauda equina results from an inadequate blood supply to the lumbar spinal roots. The cause is generally a stenosis of the lumbar canal which may be congenital, or osteophytic encroachment of a lateral spinal canal, in which case the symptoms are unilateral. More rarely, Paget's disease or arachnoiditis may give a similar picture. It may be difficult to decide on the history alone whether there is vascular or neurogenic claudication but often the pain of spinal stenosis takes minutes (rather than seconds) to resolve on resting, and the pain is often alleviated by flexing the spine. The pain of lumbar disc prolapse, which is another possibility, would be made worse by spinal flexion.

Claudication of the buttock due to a vascular cause arises from insufficient blood flow through the common iliac or both the internal and external iliac arteries, usually due to atherosclerosis. Initially, blood flow is sufficient to meet the metabolic demands of the muscles at rest but not during exercise. As the pathological process advances and the lumen of the affected vessels becomes progressively narrower, the 'claudication distance' reduces, until eventually there is pain at rest. This is a dangerous situation, since if urgent revascularisation is not performed, the limb may have to be amputated.

Physical examination is very helpful in that it can demonstrate absence of pulsation in the lower limb arteries, and can exclude restriction of the hip, pelvic torsion, sciatic referral from a lumbar disc protrusion or lumbar dysfunction as a major cause of the symptoms. There may be evidence of widespread atherosclerosis in patients with vascular claudication, and there may be evidence of predisposing factors such as diabetes mellitus. Neurological signs are unusual in mild vascular claudication unless there is concomitant diabetes, but may be a feature of neurogenic claudication, particularly if the patient is made to exercise before performing the examination.

Investigations should be directed towards assessing the vascular supply in the aorto–iliac–femoral region by angiography, and assessing the severity of predisposing factors such as diabetes or hypertension.

If there is doubt as to whether there is a neurogenic cause, a scan of the lumbar spine might be helpful.

Mr Lennox underwent a femoro–femoral bypass graft with a good result, and was back playing golf within 6 months.

FURTHER READING

Cooke E 1995 Current thinking on peripheral vascular disease. Practitioner 239: 120–124

Housley E, Leng G C, Donnan P T, Fowkes F G 1993 Physical activity and risk of peripheral vascular disease in the general population: Edinburgh Artery Study. Journal of Epidemiology and Community Health 47: 475–480

Study objectives

After studying this case with its associated activities and questions, you should have a reasonable knowledge of the following areas:

1. Surface anatomy of structures in the neck
2. Structure of the cervical vertebrae
3. Movements between individual cervical vertebrae
4. Movements of the neck as a whole
5. Testing active and passive neck movements
6. Palpating movements between individual cervical vertebrae
7. Structure of intervertebral discs
8. Attachments, actions, blood and nerve supply of muscles that move the neck
9. Testing muscles that move the neck
10. Nerves of cervical region
11. Coverings of nerves and their roots
12. Testing stretch reflexes
13. Physiology of stretch reflexes
14. Postural reflexes
15. Interaction of the neck, the eye and the ear in the maintenance of posture
16. Sympathetic nerves in the neck
17. Effects of sympathetic stimulation in the body
18. Normal physiology of blood pressure control by the nervous system, kidneys, microcirculation and hormones
19. How to measure the systemic arterial blood pressure
20. Factors affecting the measurement of blood pressure
21. Variability of blood pressure in a population
22. Causes of hypertension and the physical signs associated with these causes
23. Risk factors for hypertension

24. Pathology of blood vessels in hypertension
25. Complications of hypertension and the physical signs associated with these complications
26. Pharmacology of drugs used to treat hypertension, and their side-effects of particular relevance to manual therapists
27. Role of the manual therapist in the management of a patient with hypertension.

Background

Priscilla Morrison, a 40-year-old housewife, consulted you for a medical report detailing injuries received as a result of a road traffic accident which had occurred 2 months previously. She was the passenger in a stationary car when a milk lorry hit the car in the rear. The impact was not severe, but Mrs Morrison had experienced some neck pains immediately after the accident and these had not resolved. In the Casualty department immediately following the accident, an X-ray of the neck showed no abnormality and she was given some painkillers and a collar. There was no other site of pain. In the past, Mrs Morrison had enjoyed very good health and had not visited her general practitioner for at least 15 years. She had two healthy children, and the only problem she had experienced with the pregnancies was a mild degree of ankle swelling which had necessitated a stay in bed for a couple of weeks. She was a non-smoker, drank very little alcohol and was on no regular medication. General enquiry revealed no symptoms of any note at all.

Questions for discussion

- Is there anything in the history which alerts you?
- What examination would you perform?

Road traffic accidents are very common, and injuries resulting from the acceleration and deceleration of the body after impact are commonly referred to as 'whiplash' injuries. In this case, we are going to concentrate on a consideration of the neck, although most manual therapists will agree that this type of injury involves an insult to the body as a whole, resulting in reflexes that may affect most organ systems. Proper evaluation of such a patient will therefore include a thorough examination and history with particular emphasis being placed on an accurate history of the accident to determine whether forward/backward, side-to-side, rotational or compressive forces were involved, in order to determine the tissues injured.

You will need your partner to have bare head, neck and shoulders for the first activity.

Activity 4.1

▶ Identify the following structures on your partner:
 — Sternal notch
 — Manubrium sterni
 — Sternoclavicular joint
 — Clavicle
 — Sternocleidomastoid muscle
 — Trachea
 — Thyroid cartilage
 — Hyoid bone
 — Pulsation of the carotid artery
 — Mastoid process
 — Tip of lateral mass of the atlas
 — Superior nuchal line
 — Trapezius muscle
 — External occipital protuberance
 — Vertebra prominens (7th cervical vertebra).

Activity 4.2

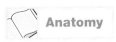 **Anatomy**

▶ Study the structures that make up the cervical spine. Note in particular the following structures, all of which are capable of transmitting pain impulses:

— Anterior longitudinal ligament
— Intervertebral disc
— Posterior longitudinal ligament
— Nerve root dura
— Facet joint capsule
— Intervertebral ligaments
— Muscles of flexion and extension.

Question for discussion

■ Try to analyse how some of these structures might be damaged in a 'whiplash' injury.

Activity 4.3

 Biomechanics / anatomy

▶ Study the details of the functional anatomy of the cervical spine. Note the following:
— How the cervical spine is divided functionally into upper and lower segments at the inferior border of the atlas (C2)
— The movements available between the individual vertebrae, and how they are constrained by
  – the angle of the facet joints
  – the intervertebral discs
  – the ligaments
  – the muscles
  – the joint capsules
— Rotation and side-bending must occur simultaneously
— The muscles of the neck can be divided functionally into those that move the head on the spine (capital movers) and those that move the entire cervical spine (cervical movers).

Question for discussion

■ Which muscles are capital movers and which are cervical movers?

Activity 4.4

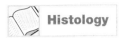 **Histology**

▶ Look at the structure of an intervertebral disc. Note the annulus and nucleus. Look at the arrangement of the collagen fibres in the lamellae (layers) in the annulus.

Questions for discussion

■ How does the disc receive its nutrition?

■ How does the arrangement of collagen fibres in the disc influence intervertebral movement?

Activity 4.5

▶ Look at your partner's head and neck from the side. Does the neck curve at all? If so does it curve backwards or forwards?

▶ Ask your partner to flex the neck. Does the chin reach the chest?

▶ Ask your partner to extend the neck. What angle does the face make with the horizontal plane?

▶ While your partner is flexing and extending the neck, palpate the movement of the vertebra prominens. What happens to it during flexion? during extension?

▶ Now look at your partner's head and neck from the front. Is the head tilted at all? If so, can you think why this may be?

▶ Ask your partner to tilt the head to one side and then to the other side.

▶ Finally, ask your partner to rotate the head round towards the right shoulder and then the left shoulder.

▶ Measure the angle that the head moves for each of these movements.

▶ While your partner is rotating the neck, palpate the movements of the lateral mass of the atlas. What happens to the left mass as the neck is rotated to the left? to the right?

▶ Now ask your partner to repeat each of these movements while you resist the movement with your hand. Note how the muscles involved stand out while they are contracting.

Questions for discussion

■ Which muscles are responsible for the individual movements?
■ What is their blood supply?
■ What is their nerve supply?
■ Which nerve roots are responsible for the individual movements?

Activity 4.6

▶ Ask your partner to lie supine on a treatment couch (or table). Stand at the head end. Slide your fingers into the sulcus between the occiput and the atlas. Ask your partner to flex and extend his head slowly (just the head, not the whole neck), while you palpate the symmetry of movement by feeling the depth of the sulcus.

▶ Now palpate the tips of the transverse processes of the atlas. Flex the head fully on the neck and rotate it fully in each direction, noting whether the freedom of rotation is symmetrical.

▶ Slide your fingers down to palpate the lateral masses of one of the lower cervical vertebrae (say C5). With your fingers, push the lateral mass from side to side, noting whether the ease of movement is symmetrical.

▶ Finally, flex your partner's head slightly, push your abdomen against the top of his head and cup his occiput in your hands. Push the head directly from side to side (this is known as translation).

Question for discussion

■ Which movements have you been testing?

Activity 4.7

▶ You will need a reflex hammer for this activity. Ask your partner to lie supine and relax. Lift one of his knees up from behind the knee so that his foot is just off the couch or floor. With the reflex hammer, give the patellar tendon a sharp tap just below the patella. Note the movement of the lower leg.

▶ Now ask your partner to hold his hands together in front of him and pull laterally with each arm. Repeat the tapping of the patellar tendon. Is there any difference in the vigour of the response?

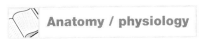

Anatomy / physiology

▶ Look at the muscle stretch reflex. Note the importance of:
— Muscle spindles
— Intrafusal muscle fibres
— Type Ia and type II nerve fibres from primary and secondary endings
— Connections in the spinal cord
— α-motor neurones
— Extrafusal muscle fibres
— γ-motor neurones
— Ib nerve fibres
— Golgi tendon organs.

There is a *dynamic* stretch reflex which operates while the muscle is lengthening (i.e. it is sensitive to the rate of change of muscle length), and a *static* reflex which is sensitive to the actual muscle length. So a rapid stretch (e.g. during a 'whiplash') will give rise to a stronger contraction than a slow stretch.

There is also a *negative* stretch reflex, which operates to relax a muscle if it is suddenly shortened. Note that the reflex initiated by the Golgi tendon organ is inhibitory to the muscles. This reflex only comes into operation when the tension on the muscle becomes extreme, and therefore is probably a protective reflex to prevent tearing of the muscle.

A further feature is there may be a direct connection between nerve fibres of the sympathetic nervous system and the intrafusal muscle fibres of the muscle spindle. These fibres appear to have similar effects to those of the γ-motor neurones.

Questions for discussion

■ Which stretch reflexes other than the knee jerk are tested clinically?
■ What information can be obtained by testing the stretch reflexes such as the knee jerk?
■ Discuss how chronic anxiety might cause a sustained muscle contraction via the mechanisms outlined above.

Activity 4.8

▶ Ask your partner to stand in front of you. Now give him a push in the back, sufficiently firm to unbalance him. Note how his posture reacts to this sudden force. Unless you have pushed very hard, your partner will not fall over.

▶ Now stand a pencil upright and give it a gentle push. It falls over. The reason why your partner does not fall is that there is a series of postural reflexes that automatically come into play when equilibrium is disturbed.

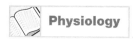 **Physiology**

▶ Study some aspects of the reflexes involved in posture. Note particularly the following spinal reflexes and mechanisms:
   — Positive supporting reaction
   — Righting reflexes
   — Reciprocal innervation.

An animal that has had its spinal cord transected experimentally still exhibits many reflexes associated with posture. In the intact animal, these are modified by neural influences from the higher centres.

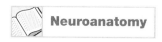 **Neuroanatomy**

▶ Study the locations of the reticular system in the pons and medulla oblongata of the brain stem.

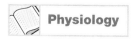 **Physiology**

▶ Study the antagonism between the pontine reticular nuclei, which transmit excitatory signals to the antigravity muscles, and the medullary reticular nuclei which transmit inhibitory signals to the same muscles.

Activity 4.9

▶ Think about the last time that you were at a tennis match, or were in a train watching the scenery, or were watching a fast-moving object go by. Did you make a conscious decision to move your head to watch the object, or did your head follow the eye movements?

Activity 4.10

▶ Fix your gaze on an object near you. Now suddenly rotate your head about 45° to the right and to the left, while continuing to look at the object. Now flex and extend your head quickly, again continuing to look at the object. Did you manage to maintain the object in focus while you moved your head?

Activity 4.11

▶ If you know somebody who has had an infection of the middle ear, ask the person what symptoms were experienced. You may find that there was dizziness on movement, particularly when getting out of bed in the mornings.

Activity 4.12

▶ Ask your partner to stand in front of you. Now ask him to turn through 360° quickly. Ask him to repeat this four or five times (make sure that he does not fall over!).

▶ If you have a revolving chair, ask your partner to sit in it, and then rotate the chair quickly for four or five complete revolutions.

▶ Now look at your partner's eyes. What are they doing? Ask your partner to describe his feelings when he stops rotating. Does he feel that the room is rotating?

Activity 4.13

▶ Many of the activities of newborn babies appear to be mainly reflex in nature. If you do not know anyone who has a newborn baby, you might try asking at your local maternity hospital if you can observe the midwife or doctor performing some tests on a baby.

There are many tests of motor function that may be carried out on babies. The most useful reflexes for you to observe are the Moro reflex, the tonic neck reflex, and the reflex which makes the newborn baby's head turn towards the light.

The Moro reflex. This involves placing the palm of the doctor's hand behind the baby's head and raising the head by about 3 cm. The doctor's hand is then rapidly lowered by about 3 cm. The sudden movement of the neck produces a reflex abduction and extension of the arms, followed by adduction of the arms across the chest. This reflex disappears by about 3 months.

The tonic neck reflex. The head of the supine baby is turned to one side. The reflex response involves extension of the arm and leg on the side to which the head is turned, and flexion of the opposite knee and elbow. This reflex disappears at about 2 months.

Head turning to light. If a bright light is shone to one side of the supine baby, the head will turn towards the light.

Activity 4.14

▶ Think about the last time you were startled, perhaps by a loud noise, or by someone coming up and jokingly throwing a punch at you, only to stop his hand a few centimetres from your face. Think about your physical reaction. Did you hunch your shoulders or rapidly move your head out of the way of the perceived threat?

 Physiology / anatomy

▶ Activities 4.8 to 4.14 should make you think about some of the postural reflexes which involve the eye, the ear and the neck. Study how these structures are related via neuronal connections. Note in particular:

— The vestibular nuclei and their connections
— The semicircular canals of the inner ear
— The vestibular nerve
— The eye muscles
— The cranial nerves (III, IV, VI) controlling eye movements
— The medial longitudinal fasciculus and its connections to the vestibular and ocular nuclei
— The connections of proprioceptors in the neck to the vestibular and reticular nuclei, and to the cerebellum
— The vestibulospinal and reticulospinal tracts going to the spinal cord.

Question for discussion

■ How are all these reflexes affected when a person sustains a mild whiplash injury?

Activity 4.15

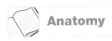 **Anatomy**

▶ Study the nerves of the cervical region. Note:
- — The ventral and dorsal roots emerging from the spinal cord and merging to form the peripheral nerve
- — The relationship of the 2nd cervical nerve root to the suboccipital muscles and the atlanto-axial joint, and the structures that it innervates
- — The relationship of the nerve roots of the cervical nerves to the articular processes and joint capsules
- — The relationship of the nerve coverings (especially the dura) to the nerve roots.

Questions for discussion

■ How do the movements of the neck affect:
- – the length of the spinal canal?
- – the size of the intervertebral foramina?
- – the angle of emergence of the nerve roots from the foramina?
- – the tightness of the dural sleeve?

Activity 4.16

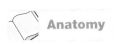 **Anatomy**

▶ After you have studied the anatomy of the spinal cord, you should look at the sympathetic nervous system in the neck.

▶ Pay particular attention to the connections of the stellate ganglion, and the difference between preganglionic white fibres and postganglionic grey fibres. Note that the preganglionic fibres originate, not in the cervical spine, but in the upper thoracic spine.

▶ Study the distribution of postganglionic fibres to the structures of the head and neck and to the cardiac plexus. Look at the anatomy of the sinuvertebral nerve (recurrent meningeal nerve) and the structures that it supplies.

▶ Look at the anatomy of the vertebral nerve, supplying vasomotor fibres to the vertebral artery.

Questions for discussion

- What symptoms might you expect from irritation of the vertebral nerve?

- What do you think is the role of the sympathetic nervous system in the production of pain in the neck?

Activity 4.17

▶ Think about the last time you had a fright, or were about to take an exam or have an interview. What happened to your body? Did you experience any of the following:
 — Sweating
 — Palpitations
 — Shaking or tremor
 — Desire to defaecate
 — Faintness
 — 'Butterflies' in the abdomen
 — Cold fingers
 — Tight muscles?

 Physiology

▶ Study the effects of the sympathetic nervous system on the various organ systems. Look at the relationship of the sympathetic nervous system to the hypothalamus in the brain. Look also at the autonomic control centres such as the cardiac and respiratory centres, and the areas involved in body temperature control.

Question for discussion

- Try to explain the above features of stress by reference to your study of the sympathetic nervous system.

Examination

On examination, Mrs Morrison looked generally well nourished and healthy. However, her blood pressure was 200/110 mmHg.

Questions for discussion

- How is blood pressure controlled?
- What causes of systemic arterial hypertension can you think of?
- What symptoms might you expect with a hypertensive patient?
- What complications of hypertension can you think of?
- What features in the rest of the physical examination would you look for?

The rest of the medical side of the physical examination was entirely normal, except for some A-V nipping on ophthalmoscopy. When you examined the musculoskeletal system, you found that she had a number of cervical and thoracic restrictions which would be eminently suitable for manipulation.

Questions for discussion

- What investigations would be helpful for Mrs Morrison?
- How would you manage Mrs Morrison's neck and thorax?

The next few activities are designed to help you think about certain aspects of the control of arterial blood pressure. You will need a sphygmomanometer and a stethoscope for these activities. Alternatively, you can use an electronic blood pressure machine if you have access to one.

Activity 4.18

▶ First of all, have your partner relaxed and lying supine. If you are using a sphygmomanometer and stethoscope, identify the pulsation of the brachial artery on the medial side of the antecubital fossa at the elbow. Next wrap the sphygmomanometer cuff around the upper arm so that the balloon lies above the brachial artery. With the forefinger of one hand palpating the pulsations either of the brachial artery at the elbow or the radial artery at the wrist, inflate the cuff until the pulsations cannot be palpated. Now, place the bell of the stethoscope over the brachial artery at the elbow and slowly deflate the cuff (a rate of about 5 mm mercury per second should be adequate) whilst looking at the reading on the mercury column or dial. At a certain point, you should hear some regular sounds. As the cuff pressure becomes lower, the sounds become sharper and then they suddenly become 'muffled' and indistinct, and they should finally disappear. Note the pressure values when the sounds first appear, when they become muffled and when they disappear.

The first of these is the systolic pressure, and the diastolic pressure has been taken at either of the other two levels. The point at which the sound muffles is known as Phase IV and the point of disappearance of sounds is Phase V. In some individuals, the sounds never actually disappear, and you cannot determine Phase V.

Your textbooks may not give you an explanation of why you hear the sounds (known as Korotkoff sounds), so I will attempt one now. Generally, sounds are heard when there are vibrations set up, and in blood vessels these occur when the vessel shuts (in the heart, the sounds are similarly caused by the valves shutting). Figure 4.1 shows the relationship between pressure and time for the cuff and the brachial artery.

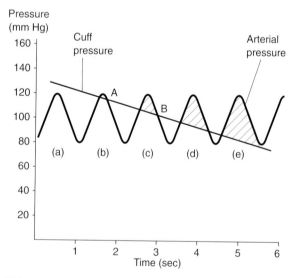

Fig. 4.1 This diagram shows the relationship between pressure and time for the cuff and the brachial artery, when listening for the Korotkoff sounds heard when taking blood pressure.

In (a), the cuff pressure is above systolic pressure and the artery is closed all the time. Therefore, no sounds are generated. In (b) the arterial pressure is above cuff pressure for a small part of the cardiac cycle. The artery closes at **A**. Because the gradient of the arterial pressure curve is shallow at this point, the artery does not close forcefully, and so the sound is soft. As the cuff pressure reduces, the artery is open for a larger proportion of the cardiac cycle. In (c) the artery closes at **B** and you will see that the gradient of the arterial pressure curve is much steeper. This means that the artery closes more forcefully, and the resultant sound is louder and sharper. As the cuff pressure falls further, the artery is open for most of the time, and again the gradient of the arterial pressure curve is shallow, resulting in 'muffling' of the sounds (d). Finally, in (e) the cuff pressure is below arterial pressure all the time and so the vessel is open throughout the cardiac cycle. The sounds disappear.

Systolic pressure is at (b) and diastolic pressure is at either (d) or (e) depending on whether muffling or disappearance of the sounds is taken as the end point.

Activity 4.19

▶ Now that you have practised the technique of taking blood pressure, you can repeat the measurement under varying conditions. First of all, take your partner's blood pressure with him supine and relaxed.

▶ Now ask him to stand up quickly and repeat the measurement immediately. Is there any difference?

▶ Wait for 1 minute and take the reading again.

Question for discussion

■ Have you ever felt faint on standing up quickly, particularly on getting out of a warm bed or a hot bath? Try to describe that feeling. How long does it last? Try to explain in physiological terms why you experience these feelings, and how the body compensates for the fall in blood pressure that occurs.

Activity 4.20

▶ Now you are going to ask your partner to run on the spot for a couple of minutes, until he is out of breath and his pulse rate is at least 150 per minute. Take measurements of pulse rate and blood pressure immediately before the exercise, immediately on stopping, and at 1-minute intervals until the pulse returns to the pre-exercise level.

▶ Draw graphs of pulse rate against time and of blood pressure (systolic and diastolic) against time. How long does it take for the pulse rate to regain the pre-exercise level? What changes, if any, are there in the blood pressure readings?

Questions for discussion

■ Try to explain the blood pressure findings that you obtain with this type of exercise.

■ Is there any relationship between pulse rate and diastolic blood pressure?

Activity 4.21

▶ Ask your partner to lie supine and raise both his legs a few inches off the couch, preferably with some weight on the legs so that he is really straining. Measure the blood pressure immediately before the exercise and about 30 seconds after commencing it (if your partner is able to maintain the position for this length of time).

▶ Now let your partner relax, and repeat the measurement immediately.

Question for discussion

■ Try to explain any differences in the results obtained with Activities 4.20 and 4.21.

Activity 4.22

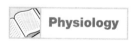 **Physiology**

▶ Look at the form of the arterial pressure wave. The diastolic pressure is influenced by two factors:
  — The slope of the pressure fall after systole
  — The timing of the next systole.

▶ Look at Figure 4.2.

▶ Compare Figures 4.2A and 4.2B. In B the pulse rate is increased, i.e. the next systole arrives sooner. This 'cuts off'

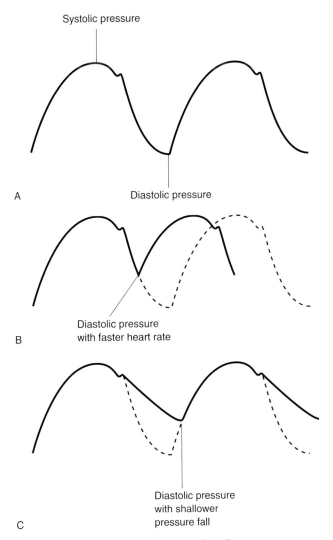

Fig. 4.2A, B, C Systolic and diastolic pressure.

the diastolic fall in pressure and so the measured diastolic pressure rises. In C the slope of the diastolic fall is reduced, and so even though the pulse rate is only at the level in A, the measured diastolic pressure is raised. (Note that in Figs 4.2B and 4.2C the original pulse wave shown in Fig. 4.2A is depicted as a dotted line, so that the differences may be seen more clearly.)

Question for discussion

■ What factors may affect the slope of the diastolic fall in blood pressure?

Activity 4.23

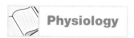
Physiology

▶ Look at the mechanisms available to the body to control blood pressure. You will find that there are several different types of mechanisms:

— Rapidly reacting – these are neural reflexes such as the baroreceptor mechanism, the chemoreceptor mechanism and the CNS ischaemic response

— Intermediate acting – these act over several minutes to hours, and include the renin–angiotensin system, stress–relaxation of the vasculature, and shift of fluid in and out of the vasculature in order to adjust the blood volume

— Long-term mechanisms – the main long-term controller of arterial blood pressure is the kidney, which adjusts its output of salt and water in response to changes in arterial blood pressure.

Questions for discussion

■ How is arterial blood pressure maintained relatively constant despite a wide variation in salt intake?

■ How might chronic stress contribute to Mrs Morrison's hypertension?

Activity 4.24

▶ Measure the blood pressure of a group of people and plot the results on a frequency distribution. The more people you measure, the smoother will be the curve. You should find that there is considerable variation in blood pressure.

Questions for discussion

■ Are there any factors that you can determine which could be associated with blood pressures at the higher end of your measurements?

■ How might a curve such as the one you have found affect how hypertension is defined?

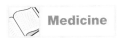
Medicine

▶ Look at the definition of hypertension. You should find that
the risk of death increases as the blood pressure increases.
The definition of 'hypertension' may therefore be somewhat
arbitrary, and is related more to the balance of the risk of
death versus the benefits and risks of therapy, than to a
specific level of blood pressure.

Activity 4.25

Medicine / physiology

▶ Look at the causes of hypertension. You should find that in
the vast majority of people with hypertension, no cause is
found ('essential' hypertension). In a small percentage of
people, an underlying cause is found.

Questions for discussion

■ How do these underlying causes produce hypertension?

■ What are the 'risk factors' for hypertension and how do they exert
their effects?

■ Which drugs may lead to hypertension? Are any of these relevant to
Mrs Morrison's case?

Activity 4.26

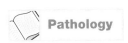
Pathology

▶ Study the pathological features of blood vessels in
hypertension, noting in particular the differences in the
arterioles between 'benign' and 'malignant' forms of
hypertension.

Question for discussion

■ How might the pathological changes seen in malignant
hypertension lead to further rises in blood pressure?

▶ Look at the tissues that are affected by hypertension. These include the kidney, heart, brain and eyes. Note also that hypertension predisposes to atherosclerosis and aneurysm formation and rupture.

Question for discussion

■ What abnormalities might be seen in the following investigations in a patient with hypertension, and why:
  - chest X-ray
  - electrocardiogram
  - blood electrolyte levels
  - blood haemoglobin levels?

Activity 4.27

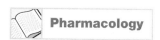 **Pharmacology**

▶ Look at the current drug treatment of hypertension. The principles of treatment generally follow the physiological mechanisms of generation of hypertension. The major classes of drugs are:

— Diuretics

— Beta-adrenoceptor blockers (β-blockers)

— Calcium antagonists

— Angiotensin-converting enzyme inhibitors (ACE inhibitors).

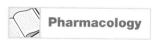 **Pharmacology**

▶ Look at the actions of these drugs. Note particularly some of the unwanted effects of these drugs which would be of relevance to manual therapists. These include:

— Increased risk of gout with thiazide diuretics

— Hypokalaemia and associated muscle weakness with some diuretics

— Worsening of airways disease with β-blockers

— Tiredness, claudication (see Ch. 3) and cold limbs with β-blockers

— Headaches and oedema (see Ch. 2) with nifedipine
— Cough with ACE inhibitors.

Activity 4.28

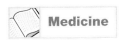 **Medicine**

▶ Look at the non-pharmacological methods of management of people with hypertension. These will usually include:
— Withdrawal of drugs which may raise blood pressure
— Dietary manipulation, including weight loss
— Stopping smoking
— Alcohol avoidance
— Exercise
— Relaxation.

Questions for discussion

■ From the point of view of a manual therapist, how would you use exercise and relaxation therapy to lower blood pressure in Mrs Morrison?

■ What mechanisms can you think of by which these therapies might exert their effects?

Discussion

This case illustrates the importance of measuring the blood pressure in every patient whom you see for the first time, no matter what the reason for the consultation. General practitioners now do this with patients whom they have not seen for a while, but Mrs Morrison had not visited her GP for many years. The cut-off level of blood pressure above which treatment is required is open to debate, but it is quite clear that the risk of complications and of death rises with increasing blood pressure.

In at least 95% of people with hypertension, it is 'essential' – i.e. no primary cause can be found. The remaining 5% comprise renal, endocrine, drug induced (e.g. steroids) and congenital causes (e.g. coarctation of the aorta).

It is important to note that uncomplicated essential hypertension is symptomless – headaches are no more common than in the general population – but once the complications arise they are reflected in the symptoms and signs. The most important complications affect the kidneys, heart and brain (NB: review these). It is also relevant to look for signs of risk factors such as diabetes or raised blood cholesterol.

The extent of investigation will clearly depend on the clinical picture. The aims of investigation are to identify a primary cause of the hypertension and to determine the effects on organs such as the kidneys and heart. Urinalysis will detect proteinuria which will lead to more detailed kidney function testing, and blood tests will occasionally show disturbances of kidney or endocrine function. An ECG and chest X-ray will show whether there are any changes in cardiac function and size, or may show features of a coarctation of the aorta.

There is a wide variety of treatments for hypertension. Firstly, the readings must be repeated to confirm that they remain high. Attention must be paid to risk factors such as smoking, diabetes, hyperlipidaemia, alcohol intake, obesity, diet and stress, as well as to drugs which may contribute to hypertension, such as NSAIDs and the contraceptive pill. Details of drug treatment are beyond the scope of this case history, but it is important to note that there are many side-effects of commonly used drugs, such as gout with some diuretics and claudication with some beta-blockers, which may prompt a patient to consult a manual therapist.

Because of the possibility of widespread vascular disease in a person with hypertension, it is unwise to perform high-velocity thrust manipulations on the neck. The thoracic lesions could be treated by thrust manipulation if necessary, and indeed some manual therapists consider that correction of upper thoracic lesions may help to lower blood pressure.

FURTHER READING

Williams A M 1994 An osteopathic cardiologist's review of hypertension: beyond the Fifth Report of the Joint National Committee on Detection, Evaluation and Treatment of High Blood Pressure. Journal of the American Osteopathic Association 94: 833–847

Williams K 1995 Hypertension in pregnancy. Canadian Family Physician 41: 626–632

After studying this case with its associated activities and questions, you should have a reasonable knowledge of the following areas:

1. Surface anatomy of structures in the posterior part of the head and upper part of the neck
2. Structure of the superficial and deep fasciae in the scalp
3. Blood supply to the skin of the scalp
4. Types of sensory nerve endings in the scalp
5. Lymphatic drainage of the scalp
6. Anatomy of the bones of the posterior part of the skull
7. Anatomy of the foramina of the posterior part of the skull
8. Anatomy of the first two cervical vertebrae (atlas and axis)
9. Movements between the atlas and the axis
10. Movements between the atlas and the occiput
11. Attachments, actions, blood and nerve supply of the suboccipital muscles
12. Histology of the meninges
13. Circulation and functions of the cerebrospinal fluid
14. Anatomy of the 7th cranial nerve (facial)
15. Testing the facial nerve
16. Anatomy of the 8th cranial nerve (vestibulocochlear)
17. Testing the vestibulocochlear nerve
18. Difference between upper and lower motor neurone lesions
19. Neural mechanisms for maintaining equilibrium
20. Connections of the cerebellum
21. Functions of the cerebellum
22. Testing cerebellar function
23. Pathways for transmission of pain signals in the spinal cord

24. Differences between fast and slow pain
25. Control of pain perception in the central nervous system
26. How to study a magnetic resonance image (MRI) of the head
27. Differential diagnosis of headache.

Background

Lisa Jacobs, a 20-year-old waitress, came to your clinic complaining of a headache. This had been present for the previous 2 months and she had been unable to shake it off, nor had there been much improvement with aspirin or paracetamol; in fact it was getting steadily more troublesome. She was not normally a person who was prone to headaches. She had first noticed the headache after a party at which the wine had been flowing a little too freely, and in fact the next morning she had felt distinctly 'under the weather'. This feeling, which consisted of nausea, vomiting and unsteadiness of the legs, had persisted for about a week but had improved. However, she still felt a little giddy when she was on her feet at work, but the room did not appear to spin round. She had noticed that the headache was continuous and throbbing in nature, and was situated mainly in the occipital region, extending a short way down the back of the neck. It was worse at the time of her period, and she noticed that it was much worse on waking in the morning and if she had to strain on the toilet. She had also had a mild dose of 'flu 1 month previously and she had found that sneezing was 'agony'.

Questions for discussion

- What structures might cause headache located in the occipital region?
- What are the most common causes of headache?
- What pathophysiological mechanisms are there for the production of the pain of headache?
- Are there any unusual features of Miss Jacobs's symptoms?
- What further questions would you ask her?

On further questioning, Miss Jacobs told you that she had
noticed that her neck hurt more when she bent it forwards,
which was affecting her when she was serving her
customers. She was also 'sick of the sight of the food' that
she was serving up, and in fact had just managed to scuttle
to the toilet on one occasion before vomiting. There was no
loss of weight, however, and there was no trouble with her
bowel motions. In the past there had been no illness of
note. She had never been abroad and had not suffered from
any recent infections. There was no family history of
migraine. She did find that her job was beginning to get her
down, partly because of the fact that there were few
prospects and partly because her boyfriend was not too
happy about the shifts that she had to work. In fact, they
had argued about her job quite a lot recently, but she had to
carry on working because they both needed the money for a
house they were planning to buy when they married.

Questions for discussion

■ How would you assess the significance of Miss Jacobs's attitude
to her work?

■ On which aspects of the physical examination would you
concentrate?

In the 1940s, a series of anatomical experiments was performed,
mostly on patients undergoing brain surgery, to investigate the
pain-sensitive structures of the head. It was shown, surprisingly
perhaps, that the brain itself was not sensitive to pain. The main
pain-sensitive structures were:

— Skin, fascia and muscles of the scalp and neck

— Blood vessels (arteries, veins, venous sinuses)

— Dura mater at the base of the brain

— Certain cranial nerves (V, VII, IX, X)

— Cervical nerves C2 and C3 (for the head and upper neck).

The tentorium cerebelli seems to be a dividing structure for the
distribution of pain. Above the tentorium, pain travels mainly in
the trigeminal nerve and is felt anteriorly, whereas below the
tentorium, the glossopharyngeal, vagus and cervical nerves carry
the signals and pain is felt mainly in the occipital region.

Activity 5.1

▶ Look at your partner's head. Consider the skin and superficial tissues of the head. Compare the thickness of the skin of the occipital region with that of the eyelids. Note the absence of hair on the eyelids.

▶ How hairy is your partner? Feel the texture of the hair and try to get a feel for the coarseness. The distribution of hair may be affected by endocrine disorders and genetic factors.

▶ Think about the last time you felt sweaty. Sweat is an important factor in the control of body temperature, but may also reflect changes in emotional status (when was the last time you broke out in a'cold sweat'?). The blood supply to the skin may also change in response to alterations in body temperature and to emotional status.

▶ Observe someone if they are embarrassed; they may blush. In the cold, the extremities may turn white because the skin blood vessels constrict and the blood is diverted to deeper vessels via arteriovenous anastomoses.

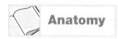 **Anatomy**

▶ Study the distribution of blood vessels in the skin.

Activity 5.2

▶ Ask your partner to close his eyes, and then touch him lightly on the forehead with a wisp of cotton wool or a small piece of paper screwed up into a point.

▶ Repeat the touch in the same place, this time (gently) using the tip of a toothpick or the tip of an unravelled paper clip.

▶ Ask your partner to compare the sensations.

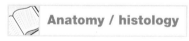 **Anatomy / histology**

▶ Study the nerve endings in the skin. Note:
— The different types of ending
— The type of stimulus (e.g. mechanical, thermal) to which each type of nerve ending is sensitive
— That an area of skin is supplied by a local nerve which branches from a spinal or cranial nerve.

Question for discussion

■ What is a dermatome?

Activity 5.3

▶ Gently feel your partner's face and scalp with the pads of your fingers, exerting gentle pressure and then releasing the pressure after about a second.

▶ Try to move the skin gently from side to side – how tightly is it bound to the underlying structures?

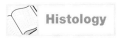 **Histology**

▶ Look at the structure of the superficial and deep fasciae. Note:
  — The variation in fat content, fibrous tissue and thickness in different areas
  — That the scalp contains quite a lot of fibrous tissue.

Questions for discussion

■ What factors can you think of that might affect the structure of the superficial and deep fasciae?

■ What functions of fascia can you think of?

▶ Now ask your partner to raise and lower his eyebrows, while feeling carefully just above the superior nuchal line. You should feel some contraction of the occipitalis muscle. This is because the occipitalis and frontalis muscles are connected via an aponeurosis, which is an expanded tendon.

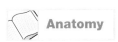 **Anatomy**

▶ Look at the layer of loose connective tissue under the aponeurosis, which allows it to move relative to the bone.

Activity 5.4

▶ On your partner's head, identify the following structures:
  — External occipital protuberance
  — Superior nuchal line
  — Mastoid process

— Spines of the cervical vertebrae
— Transverse process of atlas
— Vertebra prominens
— Line of the lambdoid (parieto-occipital) suture
— Trapezius muscle.

Activity 5.5

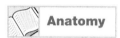 **Anatomy**

▶ Take a skull with its cap in place, or use your textbook. Identify on the posterior aspect of the exterior of the skull the following features:
— Occipital, parietal and temporal bones
— Foramen magnum
— Lambda
— Parieto-occipital suture
— Superior and inferior nuchal lines
— Occipital condyles
— Mastoid process
— Hypoglossal canal
— External auditory meatus
— Sagittal suture.

Activity 5.6

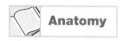 **Anatomy**

▶ Now look at the interior of the skull (again concentrating on the posterior aspect). Identify the following structures:
— Posterior cranial fossa
— Internal acoustic meatus
— Jugular foramen
— Hypoglossal canal
— Groove for transverse sinus
— Groove for sigmoid sinus
— Groove (on skull cap) for superior sagittal sinus.

Questions for discussion

■ Which cranial nerves exit through the foramina you have studied in Activity 5.6?

■ What are the functions of the sutures of the skull?

■ Which parts of the skull are formed by endochondral ossification and which by intramembranous ossification?

Activity 5.7

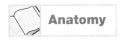 **Anatomy**

▶ Using your textbook and an articulated spine, study the structure of the first two cervical vertebrae, the atlas and axis. Note:

— That the body of the atlas is replaced by the odontoid process of the axis

— The foramen transversarium through which the vertebral artery travels

— Particularly the shapes of the facets where the atlanto-occipital and atlanto-axial articulations occur.

▶ Examine the attachments of the ligaments of the occiput/atlas/axis region and determine how they influence the movements at the joints. Identify the following ligaments:

— Transverse ligament of the atlas

— Cruciate ligament

— Apical ligament

— Alar ligament

— Anterior and posterior atlanto-occipital membranes

— Anterior and posterior longitudinal ligaments

— Tectorial membrane

— Ligamenta flava

— Nuchal ligament.

Questions for discussion

■ What movements are possible between
  – occiput and atlas
  – atlas and axis?

■ How do these movements integrate to produce the normal movements of the head on the neck?

Activity 5.8

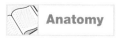 **Anatomy**

▶ Study the muscles of the suboccipital region (see also Ch. 4 for details of the movements of the neck). Note the short rectus muscles which pass between the occiput and atlas, and the short oblique muscles which pass from the transverse process of the atlas to either the axis or the base of the skull. While you are doing this, note also the attachments of the group of neck extensors to the occiput between the superior nuchal line and the occiput, and the occipitalis muscle attachment.

Questions for discussion

■ What is the nerve supply of these muscles?
■ Which blood vessels supply the muscles?

Activity 5.9

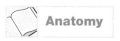 **Anatomy**

▶ Look at the blood supply to the scalp, paying particular attention to the posterior portion. Note the external carotid artery and its posterior auricular and occipital branches and note particularly the anastomosis between the occipital artery and the deep cervical artery which branches from the subclavian artery.

Question for discussion

■ Why does a cut to the scalp bleed profusely?

Activity 5.10

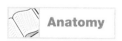 **Anatomy**

▶ Look at the venous drainage of the posterior aspect of the scalp. Define the course of the external jugular vein and study its tributaries from the posterior auricular and posterior external jugular veins. Note particularly that the occipital vein pierces the fascia covering the trapezius muscle and joins the vertebral vein which drains much of the posterior aspects of the scalp as well as most of the structures of the neck region.

Question for discussion

■ Compare the areas supplied by the vertebral artery with the areas drained by the vertebral vein.

Activity 5.11

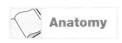 Anatomy

▶ Have you ever had a sore throat and had some 'glands up' in the neck? If you have, you will know that the doctor may have felt your neck and that it felt tender. Look at the lymph nodes and vessels of the neck and head. The superficial vessels generally accompany the superficial veins and drain into groups of lymph nodes around the upper end of the deep cervical fascia. Note particularly the occipital and mastoid nodes draining into the upper and lower deep cervical nodes.

Activity 5.12

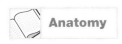 Anatomy

▶ In Activity 5.2 you tested the sensation of your partner's face. Look now at the nerves supplying the head and neck with cutaneous sensation. Note:

— That the anterior part of the skull, and face down to under the chin, are supplied by the branches of the trigeminal nerve

— The areas of innervation of the greater and lesser occipital nerves and the greater auricular nerve

— That the first cervical nerve has no cutaneous contribution from the posterior primary rami.

Activity 5.13

▶ Now that you have studied some of the structures on the exterior of the skull, it is time to turn back to examining its interior. Look back at Activity 5.6 and revise the bony structures that you found there.

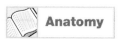 **Anatomy**

▶ Concentrate on some of the structures in the posterior part of the skull. Look at the tentorium cerebelli which separates the cerebellum from the occipital lobes of the cerebral hemispheres, and its attachments to the occipital and temporal bones and to the sphenoidal clinoid processes. The tentorium is made of dura mater, which is the outer, tough, fibrous layer of the meninges.

▶ Look at the extradural space and branches of the middle meningeal artery which lie in this space.

▶ Look at the venous sinuses, particularly the transverse sinus and the straight sinus within the tentorium cerebelli.

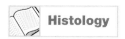 **Histology**

▶ Look at the structure of the meninges. Note the fibrous dura mater, the arachnoid mater and vascular pia mater.

Questions for discussion

■ What are the subarachnoid and subdural spaces?
■ In which spaces do the intracranial vessels lie?

Activity 5.14

▶ Now study the circulation of the cerebrospinal fluid (CSF). It is formed in the choroid plexuses and secreted into series of ventricles, which are linked together. Note particularly the small opening between the 3rd and 4th ventricles, and the fact that CSF circulates all the way down the spinal cord.

Questions for discussion

■ What functions of cerebrospinal fluid can you think of?

- How could you measure the CSF pressure in a living human, and why might you do so?
- How does the CSF return to the general circulation?
- What is meant by 'raised intracranial pressure', and what signs and symptoms may it produce?

Examination

On examination, Miss Jacobs's temperature, pulse and blood pressure were normal. There were no abnormalities detected in the cardiovascular and respiratory systems. Abdominal examination was normal. The main abnormalities were in the nervous system, where there was a slight weakness of smile and raising of the eyebrows on the right side, and clumsiness of finger–nose testing in the right arm. Examination of the neck showed a painful limitation of flexion and a severe degree of restriction of movement in the right atlanto-occipital joint. There was mild unsteadiness on the feet and a slight tendency to veer to the right on walking. Ophthalmoscopic examination was normal.

Questions for discussion

- How has the physical examination affected your list of diagnostic possibilities?
- What investigations might be helpful for Miss Jacobs?

Activity 5.15

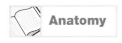 **Anatomy**

▶ In the next couple of activities, you are going to be doing some clinical testing of some of the cranial nerves. Before you do this, it would be useful for you to find out what a cranial nerve actually is.

Questions for discussion

- How many pairs of cranial nerves are there?
- Which cranial nerves contain somatic motor, somatic sensory, visceral motor or visceral sensory nerve fibres?

Activity 5.16

▶ Ask your partner to raise his eyebrows. Most people cannot raise each eyebrow separately, but if your partner is one of those who can, ask him to raise them together. Note if the furrows are symmetrical on left and right sides.

▶ Ask him to squeeze his eyes shut as tightly as he can. Note if the eyelashes are showing more on one side.

▶ Try to gently raise one eyelid and note if it is easier on one side.

▶ Now ask your partner to smile. Note whether the teeth show symmetrically.

▶ Ask your partner to 'blow out' his cheeks, and gently prod each cheek in turn to see whether the tension is equal in both cheeks.

▶ Now check whether your partner's eyes are moist with fluid from the lachrymal duct.

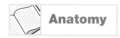 **Anatomy**

▶ Give your partner a sweet to suck, and ask him to open his mouth and lift up his tongue. Check whether saliva pours out from both submandibular ducts (check your textbook to see where they emerge in the mouth).

Questions for discussion

■ What is the difference between an upper motor neurone lesion and a lower motor neurone lesion?

■ Does Miss Jacobs have an upper or lower motor neurone lesion of the facial nerve?

■ What is Bell's palsy?

Activity 5.17

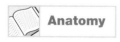 **Anatomy**

▶ Study the course of the facial nerve and the locations of the cell bodies of the motor and sensory fibres. Trace the facial nerve as it crosses the cerebellopontine angle, passes under the tentorium cerebelli and enters the internal auditory meatus. Note:

— The geniculate ganglion in the petrous temporal bone
— The right angles through which the nerve turns before it leaves the skull.

▶ Note that some preganglionic parasympathetic fibres pass to the pterygopalatine ganglion (what do the postganglionic fibres supply?) and trace the course of the chorda tympani which carries sensory and secretomotor fibres.

▶ Look at the course of the facial nerve as it leaves the skull (through which foramen?) and supplies the muscles of facial expression.

Activity 5.18

▶ You will need a tuning fork of 128 Hz for this activity. Set the tuning fork vibrating and place its foot on one mastoid process. Ask your partner when the sound disappears. Then immediately place the vibrating tips of the fork about 1–2 cm from your partner's ear on the same side. Can he still hear the sound?

Questions for discussion

■ What is 'air conduction' and 'bone conduction' of sound?

■ If there was a lot of wax in your partner's ear, what result would you get from Activity 5.18, and why?

▶ Now place the foot of the vibrating tuning fork in the centre of your partner's forehead. Ask him whether the sound appears louder on one side.

▶ Finally, ask your partner to lie on one side. You will need to cover the area around the ear with some towels. Warm some water to about 38–39°C (just above body temperature) and gently pour a little into your partner's ear. Ask him what he is experiencing.

Activity 5.19

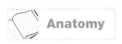

Anatomy

▶ Study the location of the semicircular canals, utricle and saccule.

▶ Trace the course of the vestibulocochlear nerve from the internal acoustic meatus, across the cerebellopontine angle, to the brain stem at the junctions of the pons and medulla and vestibular and cochlear nuclei in the medulla.

Question for discussion

■ Which artery accompanies the vestibulocochlear nerve?

Activity 5.20

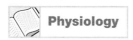 **Physiology**

▶ Study the mechanism by which the vestibular apparatus maintains equilibrium. Note:
— The presence of a macula in the utricle and saccule, with each macule covered in a gelatinous layer in which otoliths are embedded
— The presence of hair cells from which cilia project into the gelatinous layer.

Question for discussion

■ How do the hair cells signal the orientations of the head in space?

▶ Look at:
— The orientation of the three semicircular canals, with each being filled with endolymph and having an ampulla at one end
— How the hair cells in the ampulla are stimulated by movement of the fluid in the ampulla.

Question for discussion

■ How do the semicircular canals signal head movement?

▶ Review Activities 4.8 to 4.14 for information about postural reflexes, and note:
— How signals from the eyes, ears and neck are integrated in the brain stem
— The connections with the cerebellum, especially the flocculonodular lobe
— The proximity of this part of the cerebellum to the exit of

the facial and vestibulocochlear nerves from the brain stem.

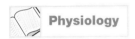

▶ Have your partner sit comfortably in front of you. Ask him to place his right index finger on his nose.

▶ Place your right index finger about 50 cm in front of him. Ask him to rapidly put his finger on your finger.

▶ Now ask him to move his finger as rapidly as possible between your finger and his nose (you can make it a little more difficult by moving your finger around slowly).

▶ Ask your partner to rapidly pronate and supinate his hands with his arms outstretched. How quickly can he do it?

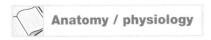

▶ Look at the functions of the cerebellum.

Although the cerebellum does not itself have a direct ability to cause movements, it is vitally important in motor control because it continually compares the actual movements (from information given by the sensory system) with the intended movements (from information given by the motor system). If the two sets of information differ, the cerebellum can make very rapid adjustments by sending signals into the motor system to affect the contraction of specific muscles.

Question for discussion

■ What clinical features would be produced by a loss of cerebellar function?

Anatomy / physiology

▶ Study the major connections of the cerebellum. Note particularly the three cerebellar peduncles, with the superior peduncle connecting to the midbrain, the middle peduncle to the pons, and the inferior peduncle to the medulla.

The cerebellum receives signals mainly from:

— Vestibular nerve nuclei

— Spinal cord (spinocerebellar tracts)

— Opposite cerebral cortex (corticoponticerebellar tracts)

— Corpus striatum (via the olivary nucleus).

The main efferent connections of the cerebellum are to:

— The red nucleus, and thence to the motor nuclei of the cranial and spinal nerves

— Cerebral cortex

— Thalamus.

Questions for discussion

■ How does the cerebellum integrate the information it receives from these different sources?

■ Do you think that Miss Jacobs has a cerebellar problem? Give your reasons.

Most of the people who present to a manual therapist have pain in one or more areas of the body, and so it is extremely important to know how to analyse pain in a patient.

Activity 5.23

▶ Using your thumb or your fist, press hard into your sternum until the feeling becomes uncomfortable. Now think about the last time you stubbed your toe, or did something that caused you pain.

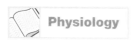 **Physiology**

▶ Study the neurophysiology of pain transmission. Note that there are two types of pain:

— Fast pain

— Slow pain.

If you think about a painful experience like stubbing your toe, you may recall that you had an initial sharp pain which then subsided, leaving you with a more prolonged aching.

The sensory receptors which transmit pain sensation are free nerve endings (for more information on sensation see Ch. 7).

Pain fibres may be activated by several different types of stimuli:

— Mechanical
— Thermal
— Chemical.

Pain receptors may be activated by any of these stimuli, but they will tend to be more sensitive to one type of stimulus. Note that tissue damage causes local release of pain-producing chemicals such as:

— Potassium ions
— Histamine
— Bradykinin
— Serotonin
— Proteolytic enzymes.

Question for discussion

■ How might muscle spasm cause pain?

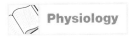 **Physiology**

▶ Study the transmission of pain signals in the nervous system. Note:
  — The different types of peripheral nerve fibre that carry fast and slow pain, and find out the conduction velocity of each type
  — That the nerve fibres enter the spinal cord via the dorsal horn, travel up or down a few spinal segments in the tract of Lissauer, and then terminate on neurones in the dorsal horn of the grey matter
  — The different pathways taken by the fast and slow pain systems up the spinal cord to the brain.

The fast pain fibres end in lamina I and then transmit signals to nerve fibres which cross to the opposite side and travel up in the spinothalamic pathway to the thalamus. The slow fibres end in laminae II and III and stimulate a number of short neurones within the dorsal horn before the signal is transmitted to a long neurone which travels in the spinothalamic tract.

Questions for discussion

- What is the role of substance P in the transmission of slow pain?
- Where in the brain do the fibres of the slow pain pathway end?
- Why is the fast pain more accurately localised in the body than the slow pain?
- What is the role of the cerebral cortex in the appreciation of pain?
- What surgical procedures are available to relieve severe intractable pain?

When I was a boy, I played football for my school. At the end of one match, I felt a pain in my foot. When I took my boot off there was a rather large ulcer where the nail of one of the studs had protruded through the boot. While I was playing, I didn't feel a thing. It was only when I had stopped concentrating on the game that I perceived the pain.

Activity 5.24

- ▶ Ask several people about their sensitivity to pain. Think also about a time when you may have had a painful stimulus of which you were not aware.
- ▶ Study how the nervous system controls the perception of pain. Note:
  - — The paraventricular nuclei of the hypothalamus
  - — The grey matter surrounding the aqueduct of Sylvius
  - — The raphe magnus nucleus in the pons and medulla
  - — The dorsal horns of the spinal cord.
- ▶ Study the chemicals which are produced by the body in this system, particularly the endorphins and enkephalins. Note that many areas of the brain have receptors for opiates. Morphine is an opiate, and is used for severe pain.

Questions for discussion

- What is the gate theory of pain?
- What is the mechanism of action of morphine and similar opiate drugs?
- What are the major side-effects of opiate drugs?

Activity 5.25

▶ Miss Jacobs had a magnetic resonance imaging procedure to scan her head and neck. Look at Figure 5.1, which is a normal magnetic resonance (MRI) scan of the head and neck.

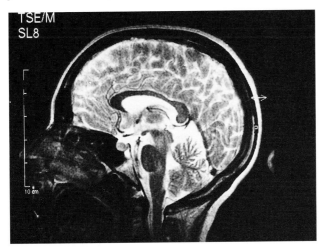

Fig. 5.1   A normal magnetic resonance (MRI) scan of the head and neck.

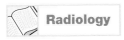 **Radiology**

▶ Study how a magnetic resonance image is formed.

A strong magnetic field is applied to the patient, and this causes the protons in the molecules of the tissues to line up in the direction of the field. A radiofrequency pulse of magnetism is applied at right angles to the original field, causing the protons to change direction. The longer the duration of the radiofrequency pulse, the greater is the angle through which the protons rotate. On the cessation of the pulse, the protons rotate again back towards the main magnetic field. As they do this, they emit a signal which can be analysed digitally. Different tissues have different characteristics, and thus the analysing equipment can discriminate between the tissues and build up an image.

Questions for discussion

■ What is the difference between a T1 and a T2 decay curve?

- What factors determine the intensity of the signal emitted from the molecule?

- How is the MRI image affected by blood flow through the tissues?

- How does gadolinium act to increase the contrast between different tissues?

- Compare the advantages and disadvantages of CT scanning and MRI. Why is MRI superior in imaging the posterior fossa?

▶ Look at Figure 5.1 again. Note that the soft tissues are well demonstrated in the MRI: the cerebrospinal fluid appears black, the grey matter appears grey and the white matter appears white. Note the white image of fat in the bone marrow of the skull bones.

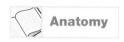 **Anatomy**

▶ Identify the major structures of the brain shown in Figure 5.1.

Discussion

Headache is a very common symptom and accounts for perhaps 10% of the reasons for consultation in an average manual therapy practice. By far the most common causes of headache are migraine and so-called 'tension' headache. Both of these are often associated with various spinal restrictions, particularly in the neck and upper thorax. There may also be a food allergy, particularly to dairy products, coffee, citrus fruits and chocolate. Alcohol may also trigger a migraine in a susceptible individual. From a practical point of view, it is important to exclude more serious pathological causes before embarking on a course of treatment. These will include vascular, inflammatory, traumatic and neoplastic disorders affecting the skull, spine, sinuses, teeth and orbits as well as metabolic conditions such as renal disease and causes of raised intracranial pressure. In most cases the history is of major importance in distinguishing pathology from dysfunction.

In the case of Miss Jacobs, there are some features which may lead you to suspect a diagnosis of tension or psychogenic headache; she is clearly suffering some degree of stress from her work, there may be some financial insecurity, and her relationship with her boyfriend appears to be a little shaky. However, it is important to look behind these factors and ask whether the headache itself, or any pathological process causing it, may have affected her mood and made her more irritable. It is certainly unusual for a hangover to persist for a week after the initial binge; this suggests that the effects of the party merely served to uncover an illness which was developing under the surface. The persistence of the unsteadiness and the dizziness suggests that there is a labyrinthine disturbance or a disturbance of the brain stem or its connections. The headache itself is continuous and throbbing in nature, and worse in the morning and on coughing. These features should lead to a suspicion that there is a rise in intracranial pressure. The location of the headache is difficult to evaluate, since dysfunction at the craniocervical junction will often give rise to occipital pain whatever the cause, and a rise in intracranial pressure will also produce frontal or occipital headache, whatever the site of the causal pathology. However, occipital pain extending down the back of the neck with neck stiffness must arouse the suspicion of meningeal irritation (from infection, haemorrhage or neoplastic infiltration) or of medullary coning, where the brain stem becomes impacted in the foramen magnum. The total illness is of relatively short duration, and seems to be getting worse steadily, suggesting a slowly progressive lesion. This could be meningitis, and although the time course would be a little long for a bacterial cause, tuberculosis could still be a possibility.

Examination of Miss Jacobs showed some neurological signs which would not be found in a simple tension or migrainous headache. There is some ataxia on the right side suggesting a problem in the right side of the cerebellum, and the weakness of smile and eyebrow raising indicates a lower motor neurone lesion of the facial nerve.

Miss Jacobs must be investigated medically, probably in the first instance by X-rays of the skull and cervical spine, although these would be unlikely to show up any abnormality. A scan of the cranial contents might show a tumour, which in Miss Jacobs's case is most likely to be in the posterior fossa. A lumbar puncture might show evidence of meningitis or neoplastic infiltration.

Further management would clearly depend on the results of the investigations, but might include surgery if a tumour were found, or appropriate chemotherapy for an infectious meningitis.

The MRI scan showed that Miss Jacobs had a posterior fossa tumour at the cerebellopontine angle. Exploratory surgery showed that this was a malignant tumour, infiltrating the brain stem. Surgery was not possible, and radiotherapy offered the only hope of palliation of her symptoms. Unfortunately, she rapidly deteriorated, probably due to a bleed into the tumour, and died about 3 months after the diagnosis was made.

FURTHER READING

Newton H B 1994 Primary brain tumours: review of etiology, diagnosis and treatment. American Family Physician 49: 787–797

Mrs Phillipa Creswell

Study objectives

After studying this case with its associated activities and questions, you should have a reasonable knowledge of the following areas:

1. Surface anatomy of structures around the shoulder area
2. Anatomy of the glenohumeral joint
3. Biomechanics of shoulder movement
4. Attachments, actions, blood and nerve supply of muscles producing movements of the shoulder
5. Arterial supply and venous drainage of the shoulder and root of the neck
6. Anatomy of the brachial plexus and its relations in the root of the neck
7. Testing active, passive and resisted movements of the shoulder joint
8. Mechanisms of referred pain
9. Distribution of dermatomes in the upper limb
10. Testing the various modes of sensation in the upper limb
11. Testing pupillary reflexes
12. Differential diagnosis of shoulder pain
13. Differential diagnosis of a mass on the chest X-ray
14. Mechanisms of growth of tumours
15. Mechanisms of tumour spread
16. Epidemiology of lung cancer
17. Psychology of people's reactions to a diagnosis of cancer.

Background

Mrs Phillipa Creswell, a 68-year-old ex-typist, had been in good health up to approximately 2 months prior to her consultation, but over that period she had suffered from pain in the right shoulder. A friend had told her that you were 'good with shoulders', and she had decided to 'give you a go'. She told you that over that period she had suffered increasingly severe and more persistent pain in her right shoulder. The pain radiated to the medial aspect of the right upper arm. There was no apparent relationship to exertion or arm movement and the pain was not consistently relieved by simple analgesics. Her general practitioner had prescribed codeine phosphate, supposing the pain to be caused by angina, but this too had failed to affect the severity of the pain. She also admitted to a recent weight loss of about 6 kg and to unaccustomed lethargy. Over the 2 or 3 days prior to her consultation she had noticed increasing weakness such that she found it difficult to grip objects with her right hand.

Mrs Creswell had a long history of chronic cough productive of mucoid sputum over many years, but she denied being breathless. She was a current smoker of 10 cigarettes per day but she had smoked more heavily in the past. She had been diagnosed as having hypertension 5 years previously, and her only medication for this was bendrofluazide (a diuretic) 1 tablet daily.

Questions for discussion

■ What other questions would you like to ask Mrs Creswell?
■ Which systems would you like to examine?

Shoulder pain is one of the common complaints that manual therapists deal with. However, pain can originate in a large number of tissues in the upper limb as well as the neck, and may also be referred from distant structures. In order to have any chance of arriving at a reasonable differential diagnosis, it is important to take an accurate history and perform a relevant physical examination. In particular, the patient must be questioned as to the exact location and radiation of the pain, since the term 'shoulder' may mean anything from halfway down the arm to halfway up the neck. In this case study you will consider the functional anatomy of some of the structures of the shoulder girdle and the root of the neck. You can refer to some of the other cases (especially Chs 4 and 5) for more activities regarding the movement and structures in the neck.

Activity 6.1

▶ On your partner's shoulder, identify the following structures:
— Clavicle
— Coracoid process
— Acromion
— Greater tuberosity of humerus
— Spine of scapula
— Superior angle of scapula
— Inferior angle of scapula
— Medial border of scapula
— Sternoclavicular joint
— Acromioclavicular joint
— Suprasternal notch.

Activity 6.2

▶ You will need your partner undressed to the waist for this activity so that you can see the movements of the components of the shoulder girdle. Ask your partner to raise his arm above his head so that the arm is vertical and the inner side of the arm is touching the side of his face. Ask him to perform the movement slowly and smoothly. Observe the movement carefully.

▶ Ask your partner to repeat the movement while you:
— Observe him from the front
— Observe him from the back
— Palpate the head of the humerus
— Palpate the inferior angle of the scapula
— Palpate the sternoclavicular joint.

Questions for discussion

■ What differences are there when your partner raises his arm in the sagittal plane and then raises his arm in the coronal plane?

■ During arm elevation, what is the movement of:
  – the scapula
  – the head of the humerus
  – the sternoclavicular joint?

Activity 6.3

▶ Now perform some passive movements on your partner. Ask him to stand or sit comfortably and to allow his shoulder to relax and be moved by you (if your partner were a patient you would ask him to tell you when a particular movement caused pain, and to point to the site of the pain).

▶ Gently take hold of your partner's arm just below the elbow and abduct it as far as possible until it is vertical. Lower it so that the arm is hanging by his side. Now grasp the elbow and push it forwards and backwards to flex and extend the shoulder joint.

▶ Now have your partner flex his elbow to a right angle with his upper arm by his side. Hold his wrist and support his elbow. Move his wrist laterally away from his body and then take his wrist behind his back.

▶ Note the range of (hopefully!) normal mobility for each of these movements, and also note any movements of the scapula, acromioclavicular and sternoclavicular joints.

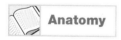 **Anatomy**

▶ Look at the glenohumeral joint. Note in particular:
  — The attachments of the capsule of the joint, and how the tendon of the long head of the biceps muscle invaginates the capsule but does not pass into the synovial cavity
  — The way in which the anterior portion of the capsule is thickened to form ligament-like structures.

▶ Study the shape of the glenoid fossa and of the articular surface of the head of the humerus. Note that the humeral head has a greater convexity than the concavity of the glenoid fossa (compare this with the situation in the hip joint). This means that the glenoid fossa does not seat the humeral head, and that only a small portion of the articular cartilage of either bone is in contact at any time.

Questions for discussion

■ The motion of the humeral head in the glenoid fossa has been described as 'gliding'. What is meant by this?

■ How does the capsule of the shoulder joint affect the movements of the humerus relative to the scapula?

■ If the capsule of the shoulder joint were inflamed, how would it affect the passive movements of the arm that you have just performed?

Activity 6.4

▶ Tell your partner that you are going to ask him to move his arm and that you are going to resist the movements.

▶ Stand behind your seated partner and put your hands on his elbows. Ask him to perform the following movements while you resist them by holding his elbow in the direction of movement:

— Abduction ('Push your arms away from your body')

— Adduction ('Push your arms towards your body')

— Flexion ('Push your elbows forwards')

— Extension ('Push your elbows backwards').

▶ Now ask your partner to flex his elbows to a right angle and keep his elbows into the side of his body while performing the following movements, with you resisting the movements by holding his wrist:

— External shoulder rotation ('Push your forearms outwards')

— Internal shoulder rotation ('Pull your forearms inwards')

— Elbow flexion ('Pull your forearms upwards')

— Elbow extension ('Push your forearms downwards').

Questions for discussion

■ Which muscles would perform the individual movements?

■ Where are their trigger points?

■ What is their nerve supply?

Activity 6.5

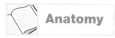 **Anatomy**

▶ Study the attachments of the muscles that both support and move the glenohumeral joint. Note particularly the attachments and actions of the deltoid and supraspinatus muscles, which in addition to moving the shoulder joint, maintain the head of the humerus in the glenoid fossa as well as close to the coraco-acromial arch, thus preventing subluxation of the joint.

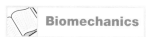 **Biomechanics**

▶ Study how the muscles of the shoulder act together to produce the movements of the arm that you have demonstrated in Activities 6.2 to 6.4. Note that in arm elevation:

— The scapular muscles initially stabilise the scapula on the thorax

— Arm abduction is initiated mainly by supraspinatus

— The deltoid muscle joins in the abduction

— The humerus is externally rotated once the arm reaches the horizontal (try abducting your arm with the arm internally rotated so that the palm faces backwards and the thumb points downwards)

— The scapula is rotated upwards and moved forwards on the thorax, mainly by trapezius and serratus anterior

— The scapula also rotates externally about the acromioclavicular joint

— The clavicle is elevated at the sternoclavicular joint.

You can see that elevation of the arm is a complex movement, involving coordinated contraction of many muscles and also inhibition of the muscles that oppose those actions. The coordination of these movements is programmed by higher centres such as the cerebellum, basal ganglia and cerebral cortex (see Ch. 5) and acts in conjunction with feedback from the muscle spindles (see Ch. 4) and proprioceptors in the joints (see later in this chapter).

Activity 6.6

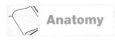 Anatomy

▶ Study the arteries of the shoulder and root of the neck.
▶ You can feel the pulsation of the subclavian artery as it crosses the first rib by palpating with your finger behind the clavicle about a third of the way from the sternoclavicular to the acromioclavicular joint (you may have to press quite hard).
▶ You can feel the pulsation of the axillary artery by pressing your finger against the medial part of the humerus in the axilla.
▶ Look at the relationship of the subclavian artery to other structures in the root of the neck, particularly:
— 1st rib
— Brachial plexus
— Scalene muscles
— Clavicle
— Prevertebral fascia
— Subclavian vein
— Cervical sympathetic nerves
— Pleura and apex of the lung
— Phrenic nerve
— Vagus nerve
— Recurrent laryngeal nerve
— Thoracic duct (on the left).
▶ Look at the continuation of the axillary artery into the brachial artery (this is the artery that you palpate at the elbow when taking the blood pressure) and then into the radial and ulnar arteries.
▶ Palpate the radial and ulnar arteries on the front of the wrist.
▶ Look at the arteries branching from the subclavian and axillary arteries that supply the shoulder area and the root of the neck. Trace the course of the supraclavicular artery across the posterior triangle of the neck into the suprascapular notch, and the dorsal scapular artery with its close

relationships to the trunks of the brachial plexus. The superficial cervical artery is higher than the suprascapular artery and supplies many muscles of the neck.

Activity 6.7

▶ Ask your partner to lie supine. Prop him up so that the top half of his body is at 45° to the horizontal. Turn his head about 30° to the left with the neck slightly flexed. Look in the angle made by the right scapula and sternocleidomastoid muscle. You should see some regular pulsation. Put your finger gently on this – can you feel a pulse?

▶ Now look carefully at the flickering in the neck, while at the same time feeling the arterial pulse at the wrist.

The flickering that you saw is caused by the internal jugular vein. The jugular venous pulse is important when you are assessing the state of the cardiovascular system. For this case, consider the anatomy of the veins of the shoulder region and the root of the neck.

▶ Study the course of the axillary vein, receiving the brachial and cephalic veins, and becoming the subclavian vein at the outer border of the first rib. Note particularly its relationship to the axillary artery and look at the nerves that lie between the artery and vein.

▶ Look at the course of the subclavian vein and its relationship to the subclavian artery. Note how the scalenus anterior muscle separates it from the subclavian artery, and the closeness of the phrenic nerve, the clavicle and the 1st rib, and the dome of the pleura.

Questions for discussion

■ Do the veins that you have just studied have any valves in them?
■ What are the functions of venous valves? (See also Ch. 2.)

Activity 6.8

▶ Feel in your partner's neck in the angle between the clavicle and the lower part of the posterior border of the sternocleidomastoid muscle. If your partner has his arms relaxed by his sides, you should be able to feel some of the nerves that make up the brachial plexus.

In fact, although the brachial plexus travels close to the shoulder, it does not supply much of the skin of the shoulder and root of the neck with sensory fibres. These come mainly from the suprascapular nerves.

Questions for discussion

■ Which nerve roots supply the skin of the shoulder with sensation?
■ Which nerves supply the capsule of the shoulder joint with sensation?
■ Which nerve roots contribute to the brachial plexus?

The details of the formation of the roots, trunks and cords of the brachial plexus vary from individual to individual. The main roots of the brachial plexus are C5–T1, but there are variable contributions from C4 and T2.

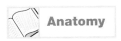 **Anatomy**

▶ Look at the general anatomy of the brachial plexus. It is probably not worth memorising the details of the nerve branching, but there are some important points that you should look at:

— The nerve roots emerging from the intervertebral foramina
— The division of the nerve into the anterior and posterior primary rami
— The posterior primary rami supplying the skin of the back and the muscles that extend the spine
— The emergence of the long thoracic nerve
— The formation of the trunks and cords of the brachial plexus from the anterior primary rami
— The close relationship of the nerves to the structures in the root of the neck and suprascapular area
— The general motor and sensory distribution of the roots of the plexus, including the root values of arm reflexes and movements and dermatomes.

▶ Note particularly that the lower trunk of the plexus lies on the 1st rib and close to the apex of the lung.
▶ Note also the close proximity of the autonomic nerves as they emerge from the upper thoracic ventral roots and leave the

main nerves to form the sympathetic chain and, in particular, the stellate ganglion, which lies near the neck of the 1st rib.

Questions for discussion

■ What is a cervical rib? Which nerve does it usually affect and what is the result of damage to this nerve?

■ Do you think that Mrs Creswell has a cervical rib?

■ What structures does the stellate ganglion supply?

Now that you have looked at various aspects of the structure and function of the shoulder region and the root of the neck, you should be in a better position to begin to differentiate the various causes of pain in this area. However, not all pain in a particular area arises from the structures in that area.

Activity 6.9

▶ If you know anyone who suffers from angina, ask them where they feel the pain. (There are more details concerning the pathophysiology of angina in Ch. 12, but for now you should concentrate on the phenomenon of referred pain.)

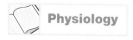 **Physiology**

▶ Study the mechanism of referred pain.

Referred pain usually arises from an internal organ and is felt on the surface of the body.

▶ Look at the connections in the spinal cord between nerve fibres from the viscera and pain fibres from the skin.

Pain signals originating in the organ are transmitted along similar pathways to the one conducting pain signals from the skin. The body is thus 'fooled' into feeling that the pain actually came from the skin itself. The area of pain in which the referred pain is localised is generally the dermatome from which the organ arose embryonically.

▶ Find out the skin area to which pain from the following organs are referred:

— Heart

— Oesophagus

— Stomach

— Gall bladder
— Appendix
— Kidney
— Large intestine
— Ureter
— Uterus.

Questions for discussion

■ Which organs refer pain to the shoulder?
■ Can pathology in such an organ give rise to restriction of shoulder movements?

Examination

Physical examination of Mrs Creswell revealed evidence of recent weight loss, and she looked unwell and in obvious pain. No position of the arm was comfortable for her, but passive movement of the arm did not increase the pain. She was unable to perform active or resisted arm movements satisfactorily because of the pain.

General examination showed no anaemia, jaundice, cyanosis or finger clubbing. Pulse was 80 per minute regular and blood pressure was 150/90 mmHg. Examination of the rest of the cardiovascular system was normal. There was some generalised reduction of breath sounds on both sides, but no localised abnormality. Abdominal examination was normal.

Neurological examination revealed a right-sided ptosis and miosis of the pupil. Sweating was absent on the right side of the face. There was some wasting of the small muscles of the hand with reduced grip strength. Sensory testing revealed a generalised loss of sensation to light touch and pinprick over the medial side of the palmar and dorsal surfaces of the right hand and the medial side of the forearm. The biceps, triceps and supinator reflexes were intact, but the right finger reflex was absent.

Questions for discussion

■ How would you determine that a person had lost weight?

- What is the significance of the ptosis, miosis and loss of sweating on the face?
- How would you account for the distribution of the loss of sensation in the left arm?
- What is the root value of the finger flexion reflex?
- How have you revised your list of diagnostic possibilities?
- Are there any special investigations that you think might be of use for Mrs Creswell?

In the next few activities you will be examining some aspects of the sensory system in your partner's arm. In a patient, you will want to establish the distribution of sensory loss in order to form an opinion about the anatomical site of any lesion responsible for the loss.

Activity 6.10

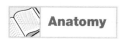 **Anatomy**

▶ First, study the distribution of the dermatomes in the upper limb.

▶ Ask your partner to undress so that the neck, shoulder and arm are bare. Ask him to lie supine. Get a small piece of cotton wool and draw out a small piece of it into a point. Ask your partner to close his eyes, and to say 'yes' whenever he feels the touch of the cotton wool. Now touch the skin of the upper arm lightly with the point of the cotton wool.

▶ Repeat this at several places in the upper arm, making sure that you cover all the dermatomes from C4 to T2. (Vary the interval between successive touches, so that your partner cannot get into a rhythm and guess when you are going to touch him. This is especially important for patients, who may try to 'cheat'.)

Questions for discussion

- Which nerve endings in the skin are sensitive to this testing?
- Which spinal pathways transmit information about light touch sensation to the brain?

Activity 6.11

▶ Now get a pin – it should not be sharp enough to penetrate the skin. With your partner's eyes closed, ask him to report whether he feels the touch of the pin as a sharp or blunt sensation.

▶ Repeat this procedure over all the dermatomes of the upper limb.

Questions for discussion

■ Are there specific nerve endings in the skin which are sensitive to pain?

■ Which spinal pathways are responsible for transmission of painful sensations to the brain?

Activity 6.12

▶ You will need a tuning fork which vibrates at 128 Hz for this activity (you used a tuning fork for a different purpose in Ch. 5). Start the tuning fork vibrating, either by striking it on a hard surface or by squeezing the prongs together and quickly letting go. Hold the tuning fork by the flat piece between the prongs and the foot. Place the foot on the ulnar styloid process of your partner and ask him what he feels. He should feel a vibrating sensation.

▶ Ask him to close his eyes, and tell you when the vibration stops. After a short interval, stop the vibration by putting your thumb and forefinger on the prongs of the tuning fork. Your partner should respond immediately.

▶ Repeat this procedure on the radial styloid process, the olecranon process of the elbow, the point of the shoulder and manubrium of the sternum.

Questions for discussion

■ Are there specific nerve endings which detect vibration?

■ Which spinal pathways are responsible for transmission of vibration information to the brain?

Activity 6.13

▶ Hold your partner's pronated wrist in one hand, and place the thumb and index finger of your other hand on the medial and lateral sides of the tip of your partner's index finger – be careful not to put your fingers on the pad and nail of your partner's finger.

▶ Now demonstrate to your partner what you are going to do. Lift up the index finger by a centimetre or so, and tell him that this is 'up'. Now move the finger down by approximately the same amount and tell him that this is 'down'.

▶ Ask your partner to close his eyes, and tell him that you are going to move his finger up and down and that you want him to tell you the direction of movement. Make a random series of movements, e.g. up, down, down (a little more), down (even more), up (a little), etc.

Questions for discussion

■ What is the minimum amount of movement that your partner can detect at the index finger?

■ Do you think that the minimum detectable movement will be different in the big toe?

■ Which structures are responsible for detecting joint position?

■ Which spinal pathways are responsible for transmitting information about joint position to the brain?

If you are a photographer, you will know all about apertures in cameras and the fact that in bright light the camera aperture is reduced. Some cameras are able to do this automatically because they have a light-detecting mechanism linked to a motor which adjusts the aperture according to the brightness of the surroundings.

Activity 6.14

▶ You will need a torch and a room which can be darkened for this activity. First of all, darken the room (the room should not be pitch black – you will need enough light to see your partner's eyes reasonably well). Wait for a few minutes for you and your partner to get used to the dark. Look at the pupils of your partner's eyes. Now switch on the torch, and shine it in your partner's right eye. Note the reaction of the right pupil. Switch off the torch, and note the response of the right pupil. Switch on the torch again and this time note the response of the left pupil as you shine the light into your partner's right eye.

Questions for discussion

- What is the role of the sympathetic nervous system in the pupil responses that you have just elicited?
- What is a Horner's syndrome?
- Why do you think Mrs Creswell had signs of a Horner's syndrome?

Activity 6.15

▶ Look at Figure 6.1 (refer to Ch. 1 for more information on studying chest X-rays). Mrs Creswell had some generalised reduction of breath sounds, but no localising features on examination of the respiratory system. Can you see any abnormality on this chest film?

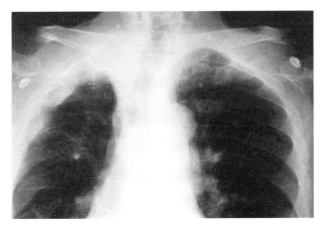

Fig. 6.1 Chest X-ray with apical tumour on the right.

▶ If you had difficulty with spotting anything wrong, try concentrating on the area at the top of the right lung. You should see an opacity on the right side that is not present on the left.

Questions for discussion

- What pathology may give rise to this X-ray appearance?
- What do you think Mrs Creswell's diagnosis is now?

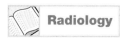 **Radiology**

▶ Find out why there might be masses in the apical area of the lung. There are a number of possibilities, including thyroid enlargement and lymph node enlargement. However, Mrs Creswell had a further X-ray of the upper ribs. This showed bony destruction. The most likely cause of this is cancer.

Question for discussion

■ How do you think that lung cancer would have caused Mrs Creswell's symptoms?

Activity 6.16

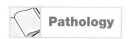 **Pathology**

▶ Look at some aspects of the biology of cancer. Clinical features of cancer can be related to:

— The primary site (lung, breast, colon, etc.)

— Direct spread into adjacent structures

— Metastatic (secondary) spread to distant sites

— Non-metastatic syndromes.

▶ Some other aspects of cancer are discussed in Chapter 11, but for this case, study the mechanisms of direct spread and metastasis. Most deaths from cancer are due to metastatic spread. Knowing about how various tumours behave may help the therapist who is confronted with a patient with a suspected cancer.

Questions for discussion

■ Does a cancer cell reproduce more quickly than a normal cell?

■ If diffusion of nutrients is insufficient to maintain a tumour mass beyond about 2 cm in size, how can many tumours grow to much larger sizes?

Activity 6.17

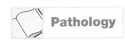 **Pathology**

▶ Study mechanisms of tumour growth. You will note that most cancer cells do not divide more quickly or more often than normal cells. Instead there is an imbalance between production of cells and their loss.

Questions for discussion

■ How do cells 'know' when to stop reproducing?

■ How can smoking (and other carcinogenic agents) alter the normal cell so that it becomes predisposed to become a malignant cell?

▶ Now study the mechanisms of tumour angiogenesis, i.e. the establishment of new blood vessels which carry oxygen and nutrients to the tumour cells. Which chemicals are responsible for the development of these blood vessels?

The blood vessels are more permeable than normal vessels, and provide a ready means of access of cancer cells to the general circulation.

▶ Note the possible barriers to the access of the tumour cell to its new metastatic destination:
— Extracellular matrix of the tumour
— Basement membrane of tumour vessels
— Dense fibrous areas (e.g. tendons, joint capsules)
— Immunological surveillance
— Capillary endothelium of the distant site.

Question for discussion

■ How do the tumour cells overcome these barriers?

One very important factor in the way in which tumours spread seems to be a loss of cohesion between cells. Molecules such as cadherins mediate this cohesion; it seems that in many tumours the expression of these molecules is low or absent, and this appears to be associated with reduced survival. Tumour cells may also interact with normal cells and extracellular material, producing enzymes which may either increase or decrease adhesion of cells to the extracellular material.

Activity 6.18

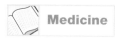 Medicine

▶ Study the epidemiology of lung cancer.

In the UK there are approximately 40 000 new cases of lung cancer per year, and the number of deaths is approximately 35 000 per year.

Questions for discussion

■ What is the difference between the incidence and the prevalence of a disease?

■ Do the numbers given above for new cases and deaths give any indication of the length of survival of patients after diagnosis?

In the UK most cases of lung cancer occur in men, but since the mid 1960s the death rate in men has been declining whereas that in women continues to increase. The main reason for this change seems to be the changes in smoking habits that have occurred in the past few decades.

Questions for discussion

■ What sorts of evidence have been provided that suggest that smoking cigarettes is a major cause of lung cancer?

■ What are your views regarding the advertising of cigarettes?

■ Do you think that smoking is a personal choice or is it influenced by social pressures?

■ What would your attitude be towards a patient who developed lung cancer through cigarette smoking?

Activity 6.19

▶ Do you know anybody who is suffering from a serious illness such as cancer? If they will allow you, ask them some questions about their illness, such as:

— What symptoms did you have which made you go to the doctor?

— Was there any pain?

— Are you expecting to have pain?

— What special tests did you have?
— How did the doctor tell you about the diagnosis?
— What reactions did you have to the diagnosis?
— What treatment did you have?
— What do you think caused the cancer?
— How has having cancer affected your life?

 Psychology

▶ Study the psychology of the reactions of patients to a diagnosis of a life-threatening illness such as cancer. There are many factors to be considered, such as:

— The patient's personality, age and previous experience
— The severity of the illness, and the nature of its onset
— The functional impairment, e.g. interference with work, sport, etc.
— The social context, e.g. support from friends and relatives
— The physical demands of the illness, e.g. pain, tiredness, sickness
— The emotional demands of the illness, e.g. preparing for an uncertain future, maintaining self-esteem, sustaining relationships.

Questions for discussion

■ What coping strategies can patients develop to deal with the stresses involved with serious illnesses?
■ How would you assess what you are going to say to Mrs Creswell?
■ Do you think manual therapy has anything to offer Mrs Creswell?

Discussion

As mentioned in the introduction to this case, shoulder pain is one of the most common reasons for a patient presenting to a manual therapist. In order to analyse the causes of the pain, it is vital to have a thorough knowledge of the anatomy of the region. The first question to ask is whether the pain is arising from the shoulder joint itself, or whether the pain is being referred to the shoulder from distant structures. Examination of the active, passive and restricted movements of the shoulder joint will usually help to determine whether there is involvement of the capsule or the surrounding muscles. Other symptoms may point to a distant site of origin of the pain.

In Mrs Creswell's case, the pain was not related to movement of the arm, which tends to suggest that it was not originating in the shoulder itself. Further symptoms of loss of weight and of weakness should alert you to the possibility of a more serious underlying disorder, especially in a smoker of many years' duration.

From your knowledge of the local anatomy of the thoracic inlet, you should be able to work out that some of the physical signs exhibited by Mrs Creswell can be explained by abnormality of the lower trunks of the brachial plexus, the cervical sympathetic chain and stellate ganglion, and the roots of the 8th cervical and 1st thoracic nerves. The ptosis, miosis and loss of sweating on the side of the face is called a Horner's syndrome, and is due to involvement of the cervical sympathetic chain, whereas weakness of the small muscles of the hand is usually due to involvement of the 1st thoracic nerve root. Because of the close relationship of the structures, it is possible for quite small lesions to produce a wide variety of symptoms.

A number of expanding lesions, both benign and malignant, may give rise to the group of clinical features known as Pancoast's syndrome. By far the most common is carcinoma of the bronchus, but other causes include Hodgkin's disease, myeloma and tuberculosis affecting the lung apex. Osteomyelitis in this area is quite uncommon, but is another cause. A cervical rib, spasm of the scalene muscles or a fibrous band attached to the transverse process of C7 may give rise to compression of the ulnar nerve, but does not usually involve the sympathetic chain.

If it is on the left side, the pain may be initially confused with that of angina, since it often extends from the shoulder and down the inside of the arm, reaching the 4th and 5th fingers, where there may also be paraesthesiae. The diagnosis may be further complicated by the fact that the pain may be present for some time before the other symptoms and signs manifest themselves. However, the pain of Pancoast's syndrome tends to persist and bear little relationship to exertion, which will differentiate it from the pain of ischaemic heart disease.

Mrs Creswell's symptoms are characteristic of this condition, and she has features of local invasion by the pathological process. A bronchial carcinoma in this situation may also extend through the intervertebral foramen and cause spinal cord compression and paraplegia. Diagnosis of the lung cancer may be difficult because the tumours are often small and located in the periphery of the lung, and chest X-ray may not show the tumour mass at all. Destruction of ribs or vertebrae may be demonstrable only with special views or with conventional or computed tomography.

Mrs Creswell must be investigated and treated medically for this condition. If there is no lymph node involvement or distant metastases, the survival may be reasonable with radical surgery and radiotherapy, but generally the prognosis for this condition is poor. Palliation, including soft tissue work, may then be of some value.

FURTHER READING

Owen T D, Ameen A 1993 Cervical radiculopathy: pancoast tumour? British Journal of Clinical Practice 47: 225–226

Palmer M 1995 Shoulder tip 'tips'. Australian Family Physician 24: 432

Mr Malcolm Grabowski

After studying this case with its associated activities and questions, you should have a reasonable knowledge of the following areas:

1. Surface anatomy of structures in the abdomen
2. Attachments, actions, blood and nerve supply of anterior abdominal muscles
3. Surface markings of the pancreas and duodenum
4. Anatomy of the pancreas, including its relations, blood and nerve supply, and lymph drainage
5. Histology of the pancreas, particularly the endocrine portion
6. Normal control of blood glucose levels
7. Clinical features of diabetes mellitus, and the physiological mechanisms underlying them
8. Diagnosis of diabetes mellitus
9. Differences between insulin-dependent and non-insulin-dependent diabetes mellitus
10. Complications of diabetes mellitus
11. Medical management of diabetes mellitus
12. Physiology of membrane potentials and action potentials in nerve cells
13. Mechanisms of synaptic transmission
14. Structure of various types of sensory receptor in the periphery
15. Signalling of sensory information in the periphery
16. Classification of nerve fibres
17. Metabolism of nerve cells
18. Types of peripheral neuropathy in diabetes mellitus
19. Aims of manual therapy in a diabetic patient with peripheral neuropathy.

Background

Malcolm Grabowski, a 50-year-old salesman, had been diagnosed as a diabetic about 10 years prior to his consultation with you. His symptoms at the time of diagnosis were an increasing degree of frequency of urination, to the extent that he was getting up at least four or five times every night to pass urine, associated with a thirst that he found difficult to quench. He had a taste for bottled water, and this was proving quite expensive. His general practitioner had realised the significance of his symptoms as soon as Mr Grabowski had consulted him, and a simple blood test had revealed the presence of hyperglycaemia.

Mr Grabowski had been given a special diet, and although he had improved a little, the thirst and frequency of urination were still troublesome, and blood tests showed that the level of glucose in the blood was still high. Accordingly, the general practitioner had started him on glibenclamide, 5 mg each morning. This had led to a substantial improvement, and the initial symptoms virtually disappeared.

He had continued on this drug regimen for about 10 years, going back to his general practitioner just once a year for a general check-up and a blood test. In the intervening periods, he tested his own blood at home using a finger prick sample and glucose-sensitive strip which he inserted into a blood glucose meter. Generally, his blood glucose level was around $7–10$ mmol l^{-1}, which both he and the general practitioner regarded as satisfactory.

However, over the 3 months prior to his visit to your surgery he had noticed some pain in the legs associated with weakness. There was also some tingling in the legs, and he had noticed that his shoes were feeling a little tight. One of his colleagues at work had told him that his problems were all due to 'tight muscles', and that a good loosen up would do him the world of good.

Questions for discussion

- What problems do you think Mr Grabowski has with his legs?
- What further questions would you ask Mr Grabowski?

On further questioning about the presenting symptoms,
Mr Grabowski said that the pain was a continuous aching
sensation in the front of both thighs, extending to the knees.
There did not seem to be any particular activity which made
the ache worse or better. The weakness seemed to be most
apparent on walking up the hill from his house, getting up
from a chair and on going up the stairs to bed, and was getting
gradually more troublesome. He did not trip up on minor
projections on the floor and he was not unsteady on his feet,
nor did hot baths or cold weather make any difference.

The tingling in the legs and tightness of the shoes were
recent phenomena. The tingling was not severe but he had
noticed it because his socks felt funny when he put them
on. The tightness of the shoes was more noticeable at the
end of the day, and he had no problem in putting on the
shoes in the mornings.

General questioning revealed that Mr Grabowski felt
quite well, had a good appetite and had not lost weight.
There was no breathlessness, chest pain or abdominal pain,
nor were there any episodes of headaches or faintness. His
bowels had been a little loose of late, and he mentioned,
rather shyly, that he was finding some difficulty in
developing and maintaining an erection when making love
with his wife.

Questions for discussion

- What do you think Mr Grabowski's symptoms are due to?
- If Mr Grabowski were not a diabetic, what would be your
  differential diagnosis?
- What aspects of the physical examination would you
  concentrate on?

Activity 7.1

▶ You will need your partner to be stripped to the waist for this
  activity. First, ask your partner to stand. Identify the following
  structures on your partner's abdomen:
  — Xiphisternum
  — Costal margin

— Linea alba

— Iliac crest

— Anterior superior iliac spine (ASIS)

— Pubic tubercle

— Inguinal ligament

— Umbilicus.

▶ Now feel for the lowest point of the costal margin on each side, and imagine a horizontal line drawn between these points. This is the subcostal plane. The transtubercular plane is a horizontal line drawn between the iliac tubercles on each side. Finally, imagine vertical lines on each side joining the mid-inguinal point and the middle of the clavicle. These two vertical and two horizontal lines form a 'noughts and crosses' pattern on the abdomen and divide it into nine regions.

Questions for discussion

■ Which lumbar vertebrae do the two horizontal lines cross?

■ Name the nine regions into which the abdomen is divided by these four lines.

Activity 7.2

▶ Ask your partner to tense his abdominal muscles. You should be able to see the vertical linea alba in the midline, the linea semilunaris on either side of the rectus abdominis muscle, and the three horizontal tendinous intersections.

▶ Now ask your partner to lie supine. Ask him to raise both knees against the resistance of your hands. Note how the abdominal muscles tense. You can get a similar effect if you ask your partner to attempt to raise his upper trunk in a sit-up.

Questions for discussion

■ Which muscles form the anterior abdominal wall?

■ What are their attachments?

■ What is their nerve supply?

■ What is their blood supply?

■ What are their actions?

■ Locate the trigger points for each muscle.

Activity 7.3

▶ Now you are going to try to locate the pancreas on your partner. Firstly, locate the surface marking of the duodenum. It starts just to the right of the midline at the level of the lower border of the 1st lumbar vertebra. In the front, this is roughly halfway between the umbilicus and the upper border of the xiphisternum (assuming that your partner does not have a paunch). The duodenum curves in a C-shape, concave to the left, to the junction of the duodenum with the jejunum; this is roughly in the subcostal plane in the midline.

▶ Now that you have an idea of the surface markings of the duodenum, you can proceed to locate the pancreas. The head of the pancreas lies in the concavity of the duodenum, and the body and tail pass to the left and slightly upwards from the head, to end at the hilum of the spleen, roughly in the midclavicular line at the level of the 10th rib.

Question for discussion

■ Can you palpate the pancreas under normal circumstances?

Activity 7.4

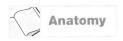 Anatomy

▶ Study the anatomy of the pancreas. Identify the whole organ lying between the duodenum and the hilum of the spleen. Identify the head, body, tail and uncinate process. Note particularly the pancreatic duct, which runs the length of the pancreas, joining with the common bile duct to drain into the second part of the duodenum at the sphincter of Oddi.

▶ Look at the blood supply of the pancreas, which derives from the coeliac and superior mesenteric arteries, via the superior and inferior pancreaticoduodenal arteries and splenic artery. Note also the corresponding veins which ultimately drain into the portal vein.

Question for discussion

■ What implications might the venous drainage of the pancreas have for the administration of insulin in a diabetic person?

▶ Look at the lymphatic drainage of the pancreas; the lymphatic capillaries begin in the substance of the gland and the lymph vessels generally follow the course of the blood vessels, mostly to the pancreaticosplenic lymph nodes but partly to the superior mesenteric group of pre-aortic lymph nodes.

▶ Study the nerve supply of the pancreas. The pancreas receives a sympathetic and parasympathetic nerve supply from the coeliac plexus and the vagus nerve. Which spinal cord segments supply the pancreas with sympathetic nerve fibres?

Activity 7.5

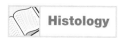 **Histology**

▶ Look at the detailed structure of the pancreas.

The organ is divided into lobules by abundant connective tissue, and there are two major types of tissue:

— Acini, which have ducts which join to eventually form the main pancreatic duct. The cells in the acini secrete digestive juices, which eventually travel to the duodenum

— Islets of Langerhans, which are collections of cells organised around capillaries. The four cell types in the islets are

  – alpha, which secrete glucagon

  – beta, which secrete insulin

  – delta, which secrete somatostatin

  – PP cells, which secrete pancreatic polypeptide.

The secretion of the cells of the islets pass directly into the bloodstream – this is called endocrine secretion, as opposed to the exocrine secretion of the acini which passes into ducts.

For this case, you will consider mainly the endocrine secretion of the pancreatic islets.

Activity 7.6

▶ If you or your class have access to blood and urine glucose testing strips, now is the time to use them. Firstly, you must ingest a moderately large quantity of glucose (the standard amount for testing people with diabetes is 75 g) after an overnight fast.

▶ Measure the blood glucose levels just before you take the glucose and at 30-minute intervals afterwards for 2–3 hours, at least until the blood glucose level returns to the fasting level.

▶ Draw a graph of blood glucose vs time.

▶ Also, measure the urine glucose on a sample collected halfway through the experiment.

▶ If you do not have access to glucose testing equipment, study Figure 7.1.

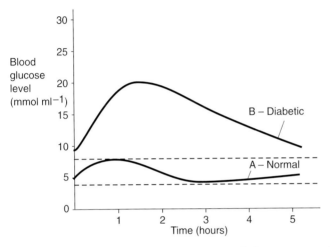

Fig. 7.1 This is a graph of blood glucose against time, similar to one you might have obtained if you had carried out Activity 7.6. Curve A is from a normal person and curve B is from a diabetic.

Questions for discussion

■ What differences can you see between curves A and B in Figure 7.1?

■ What does the Figure tell you about the control of blood glucose?

Activity 7.7

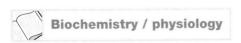 **Biochemistry / physiology**

▶ Study the control of blood glucose in normal people. Note that:

— Insulin is secreted as soon as glucose enters the
  bloodstream

— In summary, insulin promotes the uptake, storage and use
  of glucose by almost all tissues in the body, especially the
  liver, muscles and adipose tissue but not, interestingly, in
  nervous tissue

— Insulin also has effects on fat and protein metabolism,
  encouraging fat storage and protein synthesis.

Insulin is not the only hormone that is involved in the regulation
of blood sugar levels. There are several so-called 'counter-
regulatory hormones' that oppose some of the actions of insulin.
These include:

— Glucagon

— Adrenaline (epinephrine)

— Somatostatin

— Cortisol

— Growth hormone.

Questions for discussion

■ How is the body's metabolism of carbohydrate, fat and protein
  regulated

  – after a meal
  – fasting
  – prolonged starvation
  – severe stress?

■ What is the role of the sympathetic and parasympathetic nervous
  systems in the control of blood sugar in the above circumstances?

Activity 7.8

▶ For this activity you will need four plastic beakers or
  containers of a similar size and about 100 plastic counters or
  pieces of card cut into small pieces. First, label the beakers A,
  B, C and D. Put the majority of the counters in beaker A. Put
  five counters in each of beakers B and C. Tell your partner
  that he is responsible for beakers C and D, while you will look
  after beakers A and B.

▶ In the first experiment, transfer one counter from A to B every
  10 seconds and one counter from B to C every 10 seconds as
  soon as you have transferred the counter from A to B. Your

partner also transfers one counter from C to D every 10 seconds.

▶ In the second experiment, transfer one counter from A to B every 10 seconds, but this time transfer one counter from B to C only every 20 seconds. Your partner should continue to transfer counters from C to D every 10 seconds.

▶ Stop each experiment after 2 minutes and count the number of counters in B and C. You should find that in the first experiment the number of counters in B and C had remained at five, whereas in the second experiment the number of counters in B has gone up to around 11 and beaker C is empty.

If you imagine that A represents the gut, B represents the bloodstream, C represents the tissue, D represents waste, and that the counters represent glucose molecules, you should get a crude idea of blood glucose control in the normal and diabetic state. In diabetes, the glucose does not get into the cells, where it is needed, and remains in the bloodstream. This is why the level of glucose is high in diabetes, while the cells take on characteristics similar to those seen in starvation ('starving in the midst of plenty').

Activity 7.9

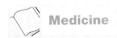 Medicine

▶ Study diabetes mellitus. You will see that it is a common disease, and carries enormous social and economic consequences for the patient and society, quite apart from the medical and scientific aspects.

Question for discussion

■ What social and psychological implications might a diagnosis of diabetes mellitus carry?

The study of diabetes is an enormous subject. The disease affects virtually every system in the body, but for this case you are going to concentrate on a restricted number of aspects. You have already touched on the diagnosis of diabetes in Activity 7.6. Nowadays, a formal glucose tolerance test such as is described there is carried out only if the diagnosis is in doubt. Usually the diagnosis is made by finding a fasting venous glucose above 6.7 mmol l^{-1}, or a random glucose level above 10 mmol l^{-1}.

Questions for discussion

■ What differences are there between insulin-dependent diabetes mellitus (IDDM) and non-insulin-dependent diabetes mellitus (NIDDM)?

■ What is the role of genetic factors in IDDM and NIDDM?

■ How may the immune system affect the pancreas in IDDM?

■ What environmental factors play a part in the genesis of diabetes mellitus?

■ What is secondary diabetes mellitus? Which disorders may cause secondary diabetes mellitus?

Activity 7.10

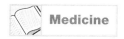 **Medicine**

▶ Note the clinical features that might lead you to suspect a diagnosis of diabetes mellitus.

The main symptoms at presentation are:

— Polyuria, usually with nocturia

— Thirst and polydipsia.

In patients with IDDM there is usually weight loss, whereas patients with NIDDM are often overweight. Other symptoms at presentation include:

— Tiredness

— Blurred vision

— Infections.

You can refer to Chapter 13 for more details about kidney function, and to Chapter 2 for an explanation of osmosis, but for this case it is sufficient to note that if the blood glucose level is high, glucose may enter the glomerular filtrate faster than the kidney tubules can reabsorb it (i.e. the transport maximum has been exceeded), and thus provide an osmotic force drawing more water into the final urinary output. This accounts for the polyuria. The loss of body water is then detected by receptors in the hypothalamus, which gives rise to the sensation of thirst. This in turn leads to the drinking of large volumes of fluid (polydipsia).

Question for discussion

■ Why might a person with diabetes mellitus have weight loss?

Activity 7.11

 Pharmacology / medicine

▶ Study the medical management of diabetes mellitus. You will
see that, as with any chronic disorder, care of a diabetic
person involves much more than giving drugs. Note how
diabetic care is organised, and note the following aspects:

— Education of the patient about diabetes

— Initiating treatment with diet and either insulin or oral
hypoglycaemic agents

— Monitoring and adjusting the dose of drugs (including the
monitoring of side-effects)

— Psychological and emotional support of the patient

— Regular screening for complications.

Questions for discussion

■ Do you think that the long-term care of a diabetic patient is better
carried out by the general practitioner or by the specialist in
hospital?

■ What would you include in an annual monitoring programme for a
diabetic patient?

■ What problems might there be with insulin treatment?

■ How do the major oral hypoglycaemic agents exert their actions?

■ What side-effects do the oral hypoglycaemic agents have?

■ How is diabetic control monitored?

■ Is there any evidence that good control of blood sugar helps to
prevent the development of diabetic complications?

■ Describe how you would go about testing whether or not good
control influenced the development of complications.

Examination

When you examined Mr Grabowski he looked generally well. His blood pressure was 140/90 mmHg when lying down but it fell to 120/70 mmHg on standing; however, he did not feel dizzy. There was a slight degree of pitting oedema in the ankles.

The main abnormal physical signs were in the legs, with slight wasting of the quadriceps muscles bilaterally, with weakness on formal testing of power. As an added indication of quadriceps weakness, he failed to rise from a squatting position when asked to do so. There was also reduced sensitivity to light touch and pinprick sensation in a 'stocking' distribution below the ankles, and reduced vibration sensitivity at the malleoli. Ankle reflexes were absent, and joint position sense was impaired in the toes.

Questions for discussion

- What complications of diabetes does Mr Grabowski appear to have?
- What other explanations could there be for the physical signs that you have demonstrated?
- What other complications of diabetes do you know?
- Are there any special investigations that might be of use for Mr Grabowski's case?

Activity 7.12

▶ Refer to Chapter 6, and repeat the activities concerned with the testing of sensation. This time, however, when you are testing for light touch and pinprick sensation, leave the wisp of cotton wool or the pin in the same place for 10–20 seconds. Ask your partner what he feels. Ask him to concentrate on the area of skin being stimulated, and then to concentrate on something completely different (perhaps you could tell him a joke or ask him what he would like to eat). Ask him if there is any difference in the perception of the sensation.

▶ Think of an occasion on which you hurt yourself while you were playing some sport. If it was a fairly minor knock, did you notice it at the time, or did it only hurt after the game had finished?

Question for discussion

■ What do the results of Activity 7.12 tell you about the processing of sensory information?

Activity 7.13

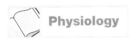 **Physiology**

▶ Look at the structure of the nervous system. Different aspects of nervous system function, such as testing of the motor and sensory systems, testing some cranial nerves, cerebellar function and postural reflexes are discussed further in other chapters. For this case, concentrate on the physiology of sensation.

▶ First you should study the basic physics of membrane potentials and action potentials in nerve cells.

▶ Study Figure 7.2.

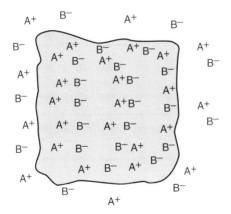

Fig. 7.2 A cell in its surrounding medium.

Figure 7.2 illustrates a cell in its surrounding medium. For the moment, just imagine that there is only one type of molecule present and that it is ionised into A^+ and B^-.
 Assume two further points:

— The membrane of the cell is permeable to A^+ but not to B^-

— The concentration of the ions is greater on the inside of the cell than in the surrounding fluid.

To start with, there is a concentration difference of A⁺ between the inside and the outside of the cell. A⁺ ions will thus tend to move out of the cell down the concentration gradient. However, as soon as this happens, there will be a deficit of positive charge inside the cell. The negatively charged B⁻ ions will tend to attract back the A⁺ ions, thus opposing the movement generated by the concentration gradient. The extra positive ions outside the cell cause a difference in potential between the inside and outside of the cell. Within a short time, the 'tug of war' between the concentration difference and electrical difference reaches an equilibrium. At this point, the potential difference (voltage) between the inside and outside of the cell is called the resting cell potential.

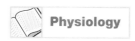 **Physiology**

▶ Note:

— The main ions involved in the generation of the membrane potential are sodium (Na⁺), potassium (K⁺) and chloride (Cl⁻)

— The size of the membrane potential for each ion depends on the concentration difference between the inside and outside of the cell

— The permeability of the membrane to the particular ion is very important in determining the membrane potential. In fact, the whole basis of signalling via the nervous system depends upon rapid changes in membrane permeability to the various ions.

Questions for discussion

■ What is an 'action potential', and how is this different from a resting membrane potential?

■ What is meant by 'depolarisation' and 'hyperpolarisation'?

■ How is an action potential propagated along a nerve axon?

■ What is the relationship between fibre size and conduction velocity of the action potential?

■ What is 'saltatory conduction' in myelinated nerve fibres, and how might demyelination of nerve fibres (such as occurs in multiple sclerosis) affect the conduction of the nerve impulse along the axon?

Once you have grasped the basic ideas underlying the membrane potential, not only can you apply this knowledge to many aspects of the function of the nervous and muscular systems, but you can also understand how other cells such as secretory cells, macrophages and ciliated cells carry out their functions.

Questions for discussion

■ What is a synapse? How is a nerve signal transmitted from one neurone to another via a synapse?

■ How is signal transmission at a synapse between nerve cells different from the transmission of a signal at the neuromuscular junction of skeletal muscle?

■ What is meant by 'inhibition' and 'excitation' at synapses?

■ How can inhibition and excitation at synapses act to cause integration in the nervous system?

Activity 7.14

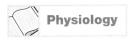 **Physiology**

▶ Think about the results of Activity 7.12, and then look at the structure and function of sensory receptors.

You will find that there are many different types of receptors in the skin and deeper structures that have different sensitivities to the different types of sensation. The main types of receptor are:

— Mechanoreceptors, detecting mechanical deformation

— Thermoreceptors, detecting changes in temperature

— Electromagnetic receptors, detecting light

— Chemoreceptors, detecting a change in chemical environment

— Nociceptors, detecting tissue damage.

All sensory receptors have the property that the appropriate modality of stimulus will change the membrane potential of the receptor. This is termed a 'receptor potential'. When the receptor potential reaches the threshold for action potentials in the associated nerve, then signals will travel along that nerve fibre.

Questions for discussion

- If the nerve fibres transmit only action potentials, how does the body know which sensations are being stimulated?
- How does the receptor signal the difference between a weak stimulus and a strong one?
- What is meant by 'adaptation' of sensory receptors?
- What is the difference between rapidly adapting and slowly adapting receptors? What might be the functional significance of this difference?

Activity 7.15

▶ If you are brave enough, give yourself a very slight pinprick with a sterile lancet. Do not draw blood, but concentrate on the sensations generated by the pinprick. You should find that there is an initial sharp pricking sensation followed by a more prolonged aching.

From your study of this case so far, you will know that the velocity of conduction of action potential along nerve fibres depends upon the diameter of the fibres, with the larger fibres having greater conduction velocities. The range of conduction velocities is about 0.5 to 120 ms^{-1}. You will also know that myelinated nerve fibres carry signals faster that unmyelinated ones of the same diameter.

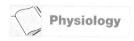 **Physiology**

▶ Study the classification of nerve fibres.

You may find that there are two distinct classifications based on fibre diameter:

— A and C fibre types, with A fibres subdivided into α, β, γ and δ fibres

— Ia, Ib, II, III and IV.

The latter classification is used more by physiologists who specialise in studying the sensory nervous system.

Question for discussion

- What types of nerve fibres carry the individual sensations?

If you vary the pressure with which you stab yourself with the lancet, you will note that a light pressure causes very little pain whereas a firmer pressure may cause you to flinch (NB: don't do this too many times – you don't want to become a pincushion). The nervous system signals increasing gradients of stimulus intensity either by using more fibres in parallel (spatial summation) or by sending more impulses along a single fibre in a given time (temporal summation). Think back to the questions in Activity 7.13. You will know that a single impulse from a single excitatory presynaptic nerve fibre almost never causes an action potential in a postsynaptic neurone. In order to cause such an action potential, large numbers of signals must arrive either simultaneously or in rapid succession. A single neurone may have inputs from hundreds of separate neurones, some of which are excitatory and some inhibitory. Conversely, a single neurone may give branches to hundreds of different postsynaptic neurones; however, a single nerve fibre is either inhibitory or excitatory to all the neurones it supplies.

Question for discussion

■ What is the difference between convergence and divergence in the nervous system?

Activity 7.16

▶ Look back to the discussion in Activity 7.7. It was briefly noted there that insulin is not required for glucose utilisation by cells in the nervous system.

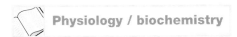 Physiology / biochemistry

▶ Study the metabolism of nerve cells. Like other tissues, nervous tissue requires oxygen and other nutrients to supply its metabolic needs. Note particularly that:

— Nerve cell metabolism is nearly 10 times that in the rest of the body

— Most of the extra requirement is to pump ions across the cell membranes, and therefore, during extra activity, neuronal metabolism can increase significantly (a fact utilised in special brain scans which can detect this extra metabolism)

— Normally, glucose is the main energy source for nerve cells
— The neurones are not capable of significant anaerobic metabolism; oxygen is required for second-to-second maintenance of neuronal activity.

Looking at all these factors, it is not surprising that if blood flow to a particular part of the brain is cut off (e.g. by a stroke), consciousness can be lost in a few seconds.

Question for discussion

■ How do nerve cells derive their oxygen and nutrient supply?

Activity 7.17

▶ Review Activity 7.13 and the questions associated with it.

You will have learnt that most synapses between nerve cells involve the release of a chemical known as a neurotransmitter from the presynaptic nerve ending in response to an action potential. Once the transmitter has been released into the synaptic cleft, one of several fates may await it, including:

— It binds with receptor molecules on the postsynaptic membrane causing a change in the permeability of the postsynaptic membrane
— It is taken back up into the presynaptic nerve terminal and recycled
— It binds with receptor molecules in the presynaptic membrane causing a change in membrane permeability and thus alters the ability of the ending to produce more neurotransmitter
— It leaks away into the surrounding tissues and is metabolised.

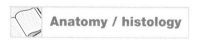 **Anatomy / histology**

▶ Have you thought about how and where the neurotransmitters are made, and how they travel from the site of production to the site of use? Look at the features of a neurone as revealed by the electron microscope. Note in particular the abundance of mitochondria in the cell body, and the vesicles of neurotransmitter in the nerve endings.

Questions for discussion

■ What are the functions of mitochondria?

■ Where are neurotransmitters synthesised in the neurone?

■ How do the neurotransmitters travel along the axon?

You have spent a lot of time studying some aspects of the basic mechanisms of the nervous system. You should now consider how this knowledge may be applied to the disorders of nerve function in diabetes, such as Mr Grabowski demonstrates.

Activity 7.18

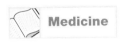 **Medicine**

▶ Study the different types of neuropathy that may occur in diabetes. You will find that diabetes affects the axons of both somatic and autonomic nerves.

Question for discussion

■ What differences are there between the somatic and the autonomic branches of the nervous system?

The pathophysiology behind the development of peripheral neuropathy is uncertain, but there are several factors involved:

— The longer the person has had diabetes, the greater is the chance of developing neuropathy

— There is delayed conduction velocity in motor and sensory nerves

— The better the control of blood glucose, the slower the deterioration of nerve function

— There are vascular lesions in the blood vessels supplying the nerves which could cause an impairment of oxygen and nutrient supply to the nerves

— There are abnormalities of transport of neurotransmitters along the nerve axons

— Some of the nerve cell axons show partial loss of the myelin sheath

— Hyperglycaemia causes an increase in glucose in the nerve cell (remember that neurones do not require insulin to regulate glucose entry into the cell); this may alter the metabolic reactions such that the molecules required for maintenance of membrane potentials are not present in sufficient quantities or are inhibited from performing their functions.

Questions for discussion

- What do you think is causing Mr Grabowski's thigh ache?
- What types of neuropathy do you think Mr Grabowski is suffering from?
- What other causes of peripheral neuropathy can you find? (Remember that many other causes of peripheral neuropathy may coexist with diabetes.)
- What symptoms might be present in a patient with an autonomic neuropathy?
- How would you test for the presence of an autonomic neuropathy?
- How are the various manifestations of diabetic neuropathy treated medically?
- As a manual therapist, what would be your main concerns regarding Mr Grabowski's future progress?
- What advice would you give Mr Grabowski regarding his feet?

Discussion

Mr Grabowski exhibits typical features of peripheral somatosensory, motor and autonomic neuropathy. The somatosensory neuropathy manifests itself as reduced sensitivity to vibration, pinprick and light touch. As far as Mr Grabowski is concerned, an important aspect of the problem is the impairment of joint position sense, which may affect the gait. Neuropathy in the large nerve fibres gives rise to tingling in the feet, with the feeling of walking on foam, and eventually to an inability to appreciate any sensation from the ground. Small fibre neuropathy gives rise to loss of pinprick sensation, often in a 'stocking' distribution, and the patient may feel sensations of tingling, pricking, warmth or cold.

A motor neuropathy often causes weakness of the proximal muscles of the leg in non-insulin-dependent diabetics, usually in those over 50 years old. The main features are difficulty in walking, especially in going up stairs, and difficulty in getting out of chairs. Formal testing will often demonstrate a weakness of the quadriceps muscle, as was the case with Mr Grabowski. The prognosis for this type of neuropathy is fairly good, with substantial recovery within 1–2 years. Excessive exercise does not appear to help, but passive movement is necessary to maintain the mobility of nearby joints.

Autonomic neuropathy is a common accompaniment of diabetic somatosensorimotor neuropathy, occurring in nearly half of all diabetics. Mostly, it does not give rise to clinical problems but when it does, patients do appear to have a shortened life span. The main problems include abnormal sweating, postural hypotension, disturbances of gastrointestinal motility (including vomiting, diarrhoea and constipation), incontinence and impotence.

There are many causes of peripheral neuropathy other than diabetes, and because diabetes is common, it is important to remember that another cause may coexist with and complicate the picture produced by the diabetic neuropathy. Peripheral neuropathies are classified as:

— Mononeuropathy – involvement of a single nerve, usually from nerve entrapment.

— Mononeuritis multiplex – involvement of a number of individual nerves. This type of picture is seen in a number of diseases such as diabetes, connective tissue disorders, sarcoidosis and infiltration by cancer or lymphoma.

— Polyneuropathy – there is a diffuse involvement of the peripheral nerves. A large number of causes may produce this picture, but common ones include diabetes, nutritional deficiencies (e.g. vitamin B_{12} deficiency and malabsorption), drugs, alcohol, infections (including HIV) and as a non-metastatic feature of cancer.

Investigation for these other causes will depend on whether they are suspected from the history and physical examination. Investigations might include measurement of serum vitamin B_{12} levels, blood glucose, liver function tests (for alcoholism), examination of blood film, ESR, serum calcium (for sarcoidosis) and radiology, which may show evidence of spondylosis or disseminated malignancy. Sometimes the cause of the neuropathy is never discovered, despite many investigations.

From the point of view of the manual therapist, there are several possible avenues for intervention in the diabetic with neuropathy. One of the most important is in the management of the feet, since foot problems in diabetes often cause much suffering and disability, and are largely preventable. Neuropathy, ischaemia (due to atherosclerosis, which is commoner in diabetics) and trauma combine to produce an increased susceptibility to ulceration and infection. A painless neuropathy may also contribute to a so-called 'Charcot joint' with resorption of bone and disorganisation of the articular surfaces. Management of the patient with diabetic foot problems includes:

— Education – stopping smoking, regularly checking their feet for small foci of infection, good footwear, good foot hygiene
— Chiropody, including removal of excess callus formation and special shoes or socks to absorb pressure
— Optimise control of blood glucose
— Treat any associated hypertension
— Recognise and treat any foot infections vigorously.

Because of the abnormal gait that may result from the reduced foot sensation and muscle weakness in the legs, there may be increased strain on other parts of the musculoskeletal system. Other muscles may be used to take on some of the function of the weakened quadriceps, and the hips, knees and spine may suffer because of asymmetrical muscle loads. All these would have to be assessed in a patient such as Mr Grabowski and treated by appropriate techniques.

FURTHER READING

Vanderpump M, Taylor R 1994 New concepts in diabetes mellitus II complications. Postgraduate Medical Journal 70: 479–485

Case 8
Mr John Ibbotson

Study objectives

After studying this case with its associated activities and questions, you should have a reasonable knowledge of the following areas:

1. Surface anatomy of structures in forearm and hand
2. Anatomy of bones of wrist and hand
3. Anatomy of ligaments of the wrist and hand joints
4. Anatomy of the carpal tunnel
5. Testing active, passive and resisted movements of the wrist and hand joints
6. Attachments, actions, blood and nerve supply of muscles moving the wrist and hand
7. Mechanics of various grips
8. Course of median, radial and ulnar nerves in the wrist and hand
9. Arterial supply to the hand
10. Venous drainage of the hand
11. Cardinal features of the inflammatory response
12. Chemical mediators of the inflammatory process
13. Cellular events of the inflammatory process
14. Systemic features of the inflammatory process
15. Principles of examining joints
16. Differential diagnosis of an acute polyarthritis
17. Physical signs of a pleural effusion
18. X-ray features of a pleural effusion
19. Types of pleural effusion
20. Causes of a pleural effusion
21. Classification of anaemia
22. Causes of anaemia
23. Examination of an X-ray of the hand
24. X-ray features of rheumatoid arthritis in the hand
25. Clinical features of rheumatoid arthritis

26. Pathology of joint destruction in rheumatoid arthritis
27. Extra-articular manifestations of rheumatoid arthritis
28. Principles of management of a patient with rheumatoid arthritis
29. Actions of non-steroidal anti-inflammatory drugs (NSAIDs)
30. Side-effects of NSAIDs
31. Side-effects of other drugs used to treat rheumatoid arthritis which are relevant to a manual therapist
32. Aims of manual therapy in rheumatoid arthritis
33. Strategies for coping with the psychological impact of a chronic disease.

Background

Mr John Ibbotson, a 49-year-old designer, had not previously suffered from any medical problems. However, he consulted you one rainy September morning with the complaint that for the preceding 3 months he had noticed some pain and swelling of several joints, particularly the elbows, knees and the 3rd and 4th proximal interphalangeal joints of both hands. The illness had begun with some vague feelings of malaise and feverishness whilst camping in Ireland some 2 weeks before the onset of the joint symptoms. He had not really recovered his well-being since that time, and in fact his appetite was diminished and he had lost approximately 6 kg in weight since the beginning of the illness.

Questions for discussion

- What are the possible causes of an acute polyarthritis? Make a list.

- What further questions would you ask Mr Ibbotson?

On further questioning, Mr Ibbotson said that, apart from the joint symptoms, he was becoming somewhat short of breath and had developed a dry cough in the previous 3 weeks which was refusing to go. He was also feeling quite tired in the middle of the day, a phenomenon that he had never noticed before. He smoked 20 cigarettes a day and drank about 6 pints of lager per week, mainly at weekends. He had been taking ibuprofen, which he obtained from the chemist, in quite high dosage since the onset of the pain, and this had helped to a certain extent. However, he did not want to keep on taking tablets which he thought were just masking the symptoms and not getting to the root cause of the problem. Direct questioning about the rest of his systems revealed no other symptom of note.

Questions for discussion

- How might the general symptoms be related to the joint pains?
- Can you now refine your differential diagnosis?
- On which parts of the examination would you concentrate?

Activity 8.1

▶ Look at the skin of your partner's hand and forearm. Note the variation in thickness and degree of hair in different areas. The extensor surface is usually more hairy than the flexor surface and is generally coarser in texture. Look at the skin creases, and note how they move as you move your partner's joints.

▶ Examine the pads of your partner's fingers and note the dermal ridges and the patterns that they form. Compare the patterns in your fingers with those of your partner.

▶ Press your fingers onto a glass surface and look at the finger prints that are left.

▶ You will need a pair of dividers for the next part of this activity. Ask your partner to close his eyes. Tell him that you are going to touch the pads of his fingers with either one or both points of the dividers, and that he is to say 'one' or 'two' depending upon whether or not he feels the sensation as two separate points. (This test is known as two-point discrimination, and the result is taken as the minimum distance that your partner can distinguish as two separate points.) When you are testing, don't forget to test randomly with one or two points, to avoid cheating by your partner.

▶ Repeat the test on your partner's forearm, and also on his back.

Question for discussion

■ What do the results of this experiment tell you about the sensitivity of the skin of the fingers compared with that on the forearm and the back? (You can also refer to Activity 5.2 for more detail on skin nerve endings, and to Ch. 7 for activities on sensation in general.)

▶ Gently pinch and lift a small area of skin on the dorsum of your partner's hand. Hold it for about 5 seconds and then let it go. It should regain its original shape rapidly.

▶ Next time you are with an old person, repeat the procedure (if the person does not object). Very often the skin of old people is lax and takes several seconds to regain its shape. A similar phenomenon occurs if a person is dehydrated.

Activity 8.2

▶ You will need your partner to bare his arm to above the elbow. It is probably better to take off a tight sweater rather than roll it up, to avoid impeding the arm movements. Identify the following structures, noting the relationships of the bones to the skin creases:
— Ulnar styloid process
— Radial styloid process
— Dorsal tubercle of radius
— Pisiform bone
— Scaphoid tubercle
— Metacarpal heads
— Metacarpals 1–5
— Proximal phalanges 1–5
— Middle phalanges 2–5
— Distal phalanges 1–5
— Hook of hamate
— Ridge of trapezium.

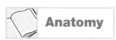 **Anatomy**

▶ Study the bones of the wrist and hand. Note:

— The concavity of the distal end of the radius and ulna, and the fact that the convexity of the distal row of the carpal bones is greater than the radio-ulnar concavity

— That the radial margin of the radius protrudes further distally than does the ulnar margin and that the dorsal surface protrudes further than the palmar surface

— The two rows of carpal bones, each being generally roughly cuboid, with four articulating surfaces and two surfaces attached to ligaments

— The concavity of the carpal bones as a whole on the palmar surface.

Question for discussion

■ What structure maintains the concavity of the carpal arch?

▶ Look at the five metacarpal bones and note that they articulate with four carpal bones.

▶ Look at the articular facets on the carpal and metacarpal bones, and in particular the arrangement of the 2nd and 3rd metacarpals.

Question for discussion

■ What might be the functional significance of the arrangement of the articular facets between carpals and metacarpals?

▶ Look at the shape of the distal ends of the metacarpals as they articulate with the phalanges. Note the fact that the convexity of the distal end of the metacarpal is greater than the concavity of the proximal end of the corresponding phalanx.

▶ Look at the phalanges as they articulate with each other at the interphalangeal joints.

Question for discussion

■ What differences are there between the metacarpophalangeal joints and the interphalangeal joints?

Activity 8.3

▶ Ask your partner to relax his hand and wrist. Place your right hand in his hand and your left hand on his forearm just above the wrist, and gently grip these areas. Move the wrist joint passively to make the following movements:

— Flexion
— Extension
— Radial deviation
— Ulnar deviation
— Pronation
— Supination.

Questions for discussion

■ Which of these movements does not occur at the wrist (radiocarpal) joint?

■ What is the range of the various movements?

▶ Repeat this activity for each joint in the hand, holding the bones on either side of the joint, moving them passively to the maximum extent and noting the range of movement in each direction.

Activity 8.4

 Anatomy / biomechanics

▶ Study how the bones of the wrist and hand move relative to one another to produce the movements. Note that movements at the radiocarpal joint are flexion, extension and ulnar and radial deviation; pronation and supination occur at the proximal radio-ulnar joint. Note the gliding motion between the radius and carpal bones.

▶ Study the ligaments of the wrist and their role in movement. Note how the ulnar collateral ligament becomes taut when the wrist is deviated to the radial side and the radial collateral ligament becomes taut on ulnar deviation. The ligaments on the palmar surface of the wrist help to maintain the carpal arch, and tighten on supination, whereas the dorsal ligaments tighten on pronation.

Question for discussion

■ How do the carpal bones move relative to one another and to the radius in the following movements of the wrist:
  – Palmar flexion
  – Dorsiflexion

- Radial deviation
- Ulnar deviation.

▶ Study the carpal tunnel, which is formed by the carpal bones and the flexor retinaculum. Note:
  — The contents of the carpal tunnel, and the fact that the flexor retinaculum prevents bowing of the flexor tendons of the wrist and hand during palmar flexion
  — That while the distal part of the retinaculum is fixed between the trapezium and hamate, the proximal part may be relaxed by movement of the pisiform, as happens if flexor carpi ulnaris is not contracting.

▶ Now ask your partner to flex his fingers at the metacarpo-phalangeal joints. Try to abduct and adduct the fingers.

▶ Try again when the fingers are extended; you should find that adduction and abduction of the fingers is much easier.

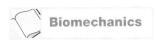 **Biomechanics**

▶ Look at how the arrangement of the ligaments at the metacarpal heads causes then to tighten during flexion, thus limiting adduction and abduction.

Activity 8.5

▶ Look at the muscles and tendons of your partner's forearm, wrist and hand. Try to identify the following:
  — Tendon of flexor carpi ulnaris
  — Tendon of palmaris longus
  — Tendon of flexor carpi radialis
  — Tendon of abductor pollicis longus
  — Tendon of extensor pollicis brevis
  — Tendon of extensor pollicis longus
  — Tendon of extensor carpi ulnaris
  — Tendon of extensor digitorum
  — Thenar eminence
  — Hypothenar eminence.

Question for discussion

■ Which tendons form the boundaries of the 'anatomical snuff box'?

Activity 8.6

▶ Have your partner seated comfortably with one arm resting on a table. Ask your partner to perform the following movements, each against your resistance:

— Wrist palmar flexion

— Wrist dorsiflexion

— Wrist abduction

— Wrist adduction

— Thumb adduction

— Thumb abduction

— Thumb flexion

— Thumb extension

— Thumb opposition (touching the tip of the thumb to the 5th finger)

— Finger palmar flexion at the metacarpophalangeal joints

— Finger extension

— Finger flexion at the interphalangeal joints

— Finger abduction

— Finger adduction.

As you can see, there is a vast range of individual movements in the joints of the hand. However, from a functional viewpoint, these movements become useful only when they are combined into various grips.

▶ Ask your partner to perform the following tasks:

— Pick up a grain of rice

— Hold a briefcase or shopping bag by the handle

— Drive in a screw using a screwdriver

— Drive in a nail using a hammer

— Write a few words using pen and paper

— Unscrew the lid of a jar

— Clench the fist

— Insert a key into a lock and turn it.

▶ See if you can analyse the movements that are involved in each of these movements. You will probably not be surprised to note that many of these movements involve contraction of muscles of the forearm, upper arm and even the shoulder girdle, but for the moment just concentrate on the movements of the wrist and hands.

Activity 8.7

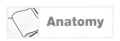 **Anatomy**

▶ Study the muscles that control the movements of the hand and wrist. Note:

— The attachments of the forearm muscles to the common flexor and extensor origins

— That brachioradialis acts as an elbow flexor when the forearm is in mid-pronation, although it arises close to the extensor origin.

▶ Look at the insertion of the flexor tendons of the fingers, with the tendon of the profundus muscle inserting into the distal phalanx and the superficialis tendon dividing to enclose the profundus and attaching to the sides of the middle phalanx. Note the synovial sheaths surrounding the flexor tendons, preventing friction developing as the tendon moves against bony prominences.

▶ Look at the insertion of the extensor tendons of the fingers, which split at the distal end of the proximal phalanx and join with the lumbricals and interossei to form the extensor expansion.

Questions for discussion

■ Why is it not possible to extend completely the wrist and the fingers at the same time?

■ What is the action of the extensor digitorum muscle acting alone?

■ Which muscles are required to fully extend the fingers?

▶ Look at the attachments of the interossei and the lumbricals. They lie on the palmar aspect of the hand, but their tendons travel to the extensor expansion. Thus they help to flex the metacarpophalangeal joints but extend the distal interphalangeal joints.

▶ Finally, study the attachments of the muscles of the thenar and hypothenar eminences, and particularly note the muscles which cause opposition of the thumb, which involves in turn, extension, abduction, flexion and adduction of the thumb.

Question for discussion

■ What differences are there in muscles used between a gentle and a firm grip?

Activity 8.8

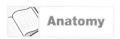 **Anatomy**

▶ On your partner's hand and with the help of your textbook, trace the course of the median nerve in the wrist and hand. Note that the median nerve runs in the carpal tunnel and gives off a recurrent branch in the palm.

Questions for discussion

■ What are the nerve roots of the median nerve?
■ Which cords of the brachial plexus form the median nerve?
■ Which muscles in the hand are supplied by the median nerve?
■ What sensory area in the hand is supplied by the median nerve?
■ What is 'carpal tunnel syndrome'? What is its cause? What symptoms might it produce?
■ How would you test clinically the muscles supplied by the median nerve in the hand?
■ What differences are there between a severance of the median nerve at the wrist and a severance above the elbow?

Activity 8.9

▶ Study the course of the ulnar nerve in the wrist and hand of your partner. Note that it passes above the flexor retinaculum and travels close to the pisiform and the hook of hamate, and gives off palmar and dorsal branches that supply the skin of the ulnar aspect of the hand.

Questions for discussion

■ What are the nerve roots of the ulnar nerve?
■ Which cords of the brachial plexus form the ulnar nerve?

- Which muscles in the hand are supplied by the ulnar nerve?
- What sensory area in the hand is supplied by the ulnar nerve?
- How would you test clinically the muscles supplied by the ulnar nerve in the hand?
- What differences are there between a severance of the ulnar nerve at the wrist and a severance at the elbow?
- Why is the median nerve essential for a precision grip (e.g. picking up a grain of rice) while the ulnar nerve is essential for a power grip (e.g. holding a hammer)?
- What happens when you hit your 'funny bone'?

Activity 8.10

▶ Study the course of the radial nerve in the wrist and hand of your partner. Note that it crosses the tendon of brachioradialis just proximal to the anatomical snuff box, where it may be palpable.

▶ Note that the radial nerve in the hand is entirely sensory. Ask your partner to extend his thumb, and palpate over the tendon of extensor pollicis longus. You may be able to feel one of the digital branches of the radial nerve. Note that the posterior interosseous nerve, which is the deep branch of the radial nerve and which arises at the elbow, supplies sensory fibres to the joints of the wrist.

Questions for discussion

- What are the nerve roots of the radial nerve?
- Which cords of the brachial plexus form the radial nerve?
- What sensory area in the hand is supplied by the radial nerve?
- What symptoms would be produced by severing the radial nerve at the wrist? Above the elbow?
- What is 'wrist drop'? Which muscles are affected in wrist drop?
- What is a 'Saturday night palsy'?

Activity 8.11

▶ On your partner's wrist, palpate the pulsation of the radial artery. Count the number of pulsations per minute, and determine whether the pulse is regular. If you look very carefully, you may be able to see the pulsations of the radial artery, but it is not usually very obvious. You may find it easier to see the radial artery pulsating in an older person whose arteries are less compliant.

▶ Feel the radial artery pulsating in the floor of the anatomical snuff box.

▶ Palpate the ulnar artery on the medial side of the wrist as it passes just above the flexor retinaculum.

▶ Measure the systolic blood pressure by palpating the radial artery, inflating the sphygmomanometer cuff to well above systolic pressure (this obliterates the pulsations) and then noting the pressure at which the pulsations return as the cuff pressure falls. (There are other activities on taking blood pressure in Ch. 4.)

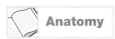 **Anatomy**

▶ Study the arterial supply to the hand. Note:
— The superficial and deep palmar arches and the dorsal arch, all of which connect the radial and ulnar arteries
— The digital arteries, which arise from the superficial palmar arch.

▶ Observe the veins of the hand and wrist. (You can make the veins on your partner stand out more if you ask him to lower his hand so that his arm hangs down, or by gripping his forearm to occlude the venous return from the tissue of the hand. Either of these manoeuvres will be more effective if the room is warm.)

▶ Compare the veins on the back of your partner's hand with those of your own. Note the cephalic vein in the anatomical snuff box; this site is commonly used for the insertion of intravenous infusions. (See Ch. 2 for more activities regarding blood flow in veins.) Confirm the venous drainage of the hand by looking in your textbook.

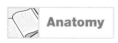 **Anatomy**

The lymphatic drainage of the hand is not visible in the living person, but generally the superficial lymphatic vessels travel with the superficial veins, and the deep lymphatics drain the deeper tissues and travel with the deep vessels.

Examination 1

On examination, Mr Ibbotson appeared clinically anaemic and his temperature was slightly elevated at 38°C. In the respiratory system, the respiratory rate was slightly elevated at 24 per minute, and there was dullness to percussion with absent breath sounds in the left lower zone posteriorly and also in the left axillary region. In the cardiovascular system the pulse was 96 per minute and regular, and the blood pressure 125/75 mmHg. There was a soft mid-systolic murmur heard maximally at the apex. Jugular venous pressure was not elevated and there was no pitting oedema of the ankles. The affected joints were all swollen and warm with pain and tenderness and limitation of passive movement. There was soft tissue swelling bilaterally in the fingers with pain on finger flexion. The glands in both axillae and groins were slightly enlarged and tender.

Questions for discussion

- What reasons can you think of for Mr Ibbotson's anaemia?
- What do the physical signs in the chest signify?
- What do you think is the significance of the heart murmur?
- What does the swelling in the fingers signify?
- What is your differential diagnosis now?
- What investigations do you think might be useful?
- How would you manage Mr Ibbotson?

If you have ever had a boil or a septic finger, you will be familiar with the manifestations of the inflammatory process. If you were in pain, or confined to bed, you might be surprised to know that the inflammatory process is not a disease but is actually one of the body's defence mechanisms against tissue injury! In general, the outcome of the process is beneficial, but sometimes more harm than good is done.

Activity 8.12

▶ If you know someone who has a boil and will let you examine it, note that it displays the following features:

— It is warm. Gently touch the boil with the dorsal aspect of one of your proximal phalanges, and compare its temperature with that of a surrounding normal area.

— It is red. Gently press the boil and note that the redness returns rapidly after you remove your pressure. Again compare this with some surrounding normal tissue.

— It is swollen. You will note that the boil is generally raised above the surface of the skin. You would be able to press on it to disperse the fluid if it were not for the fact that:

— It is painful.

These four features (Latin names: calor (heat); rubor (redness); turgor (swelling); dolor (pain)) are termed the cardinal signs of inflammation. Inflammation in a particular area often has a term which ends in -itis (e.g. appendicitis, arthritis). Mr Ibbotson seems to have an -itis in some of his joints. It is therefore appropriate for you to study some aspects of the pathophysiology of inflammation.

▶ Refer back to Chapter 2, where you will find activities on capillary permeability, and to Chapter 3 where there are activities on blood flow.

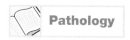 **Pathology**

▶ Look at acute inflammation. You will find the cardinal features described and you will note that the blood vessels have an important role to play in their development. Note that:

— Calor (heat) and rubor (redness) are both caused by vasodilatation, which increases the flow of warm, red blood to the affected area

— Turgor (swelling) is caused by increased venous pressure from the vasodilatation, and increased permeability of the capillary walls

— Dolor (pain) is produced by mechanical stretching of tissue by the swelling, and by chemicals that are released in the inflammatory reaction (the so-called 'chemical mediators').

Questions for discussion

■ What causes of the inflammatory process (apart from infection) can you think of?

- How many -itis words can you find?
- What possible outcomes are there of the acute inflammatory process?
- What is the difference between a transudate and an exudate?

Activity 8.13

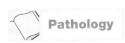 **Pathology**

▶ Study the underlying mechanisms of the inflammatory process. Note that:
— There are two major aspects to study, namely
  - chemical mediators
  - cells
— The chemical mediators are derived from a number of sources, including:
  - plasma
  - inflammatory cells
  - the inflamed tissue.

Question for discussion

- What criteria must a proposed chemical mediator of inflammation fulfil in order for it to be regarded as an established mediator?

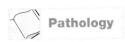 **Pathology**

▶ Study the important chemical mediators of inflammation, including:
— Derivatives of arachidonic acid
— Cytokines, lymphokines, monokines
— Histamine, and other vasoactive amines
— Growth factor
— Contents of lysosomes
— Complement system
— Clotting system products
— Fibrinolytic system products

— Kinins

— Platelet activating factor.

There are complex interactions of these factors which have effects that depend upon the severity and nature of the injury and the tissue involved.

Questions for discussion

■ How do the various chemicals produce the cardinal signs of inflammation?

■ Why does a person suffering from a severe inflammatory disorder often have a fever?

■ What other roles do the inflammatory mediators play in normal and abnormal situations?

You have almost certainly had a cold during which you coughed up green or yellow phlegm (technical term 'sputum'). Similarly, if you have had a boil which has had to be incised, you will know that a thick, greenish-yellow liquid came out from it. Both these situations illustrate the formation of an inflammatory exudate with inflammatory cells (known as pus).

Activity 8.14

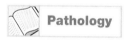 **Pathology**

▶ Study the cellular events of the inflammatory process.

In acute inflammation the main cells are neutrophils and macrophages. There are several steps involved in the movement of these cells out of the blood stream and into the inflamed tissues:

— Margination of the cells to the sides of the vessels

— Adhesion of cells to the vascular endothelium

— Emigration of cells through the vessel wall

— Chemotaxis towards a chemical stimulus

— Phagocytosis of bacteria and debris.

Questions for discussion

■ How do chemical mediators act to accomplish each of the steps outlined above?

■ How do neutrophils kill bacteria?

Activity 8.15

▶ If you have had a severe inflammatory disease, or know someone who has, consider the generalised effects of inflammation. Think back to your own illness or ask your 'patient' about the general feelings during the illness. How many of the following list did you or your patient experience:

— Fever
— Sweating
— Rigors (uncontrolled shaking)
— Palpitations, with tachycardia (fast heart rate)
— Loss of weight and appetite
— Weakness of muscles
— Aching of muscles
— Nausea and vomiting?

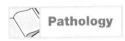 **Pathology**

▶ Study these systemic effects (called 'acute-phase reactions').

Some of the chemical mediators of inflammation alter metabolism in the liver, leading to production of acute-phase proteins, which are responsible for many of the features mentioned above. Note also that any kind of stress to the body will affect the adrenal glands via the hypothalamus and pituitary gland. Stimulation of these glands will cause excess production of hormones such as growth hormone, cortisol, adrenaline and prolactin. You will need to consult your physiology textbook for details of these hormones, but essentially they affect carbohydrate and fat metabolism and transport of sodium and potassium in cells.

Question for discussion

■ Does Mr Ibbotson have any generalised symptoms?

In the next activity, you are going to look at some basic principles of examining joints. You have already performed some of the appropriate manoeuvres earlier in this chapter, but it is worth putting these into a routine which you can apply to many patients.

When examining a joint, the important points in your routine should be:

— Inspection (look)

— Palpation (feel)

— Passive movement (you move the joint)

— Active movement (the patient moves the joint)

— Resisted movement (you resist the patient's movement).

The movements will obviously be specific to the joint under investigation, which is why it is important to know the functional anatomy of the joints, including the muscles and their nerve supply.

Activity 8.16

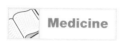 **Medicine**

▶ Study the aspects of inspection and palpation that apply to most joints. Note particularly that many diseases that affect joints also affect other body systems, and so a complete physical examination is often necessary to get to the root of the problem. Examination of the joint includes looking and feeling for:

— Deformity

— Swelling

— Muscle wasting around the joint

— Scars indicating previous surgery or infection

— Warmth

— Tenderness

— Synovial thickening

— Distribution of joint involvement.

Questions for discussion

■ What factors may contribute to joint deformity?

■ How would you distinguish a joint effusion from synovial thickening by examination of the joint?

Activity 8.17

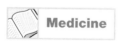 **Medicine**

▶ Study the main causes of Mr Ibbotson's type of arthritis, which is an acute polyarthritis.

There is quite a wide differential diagnosis of disorders which may present as an acute polyarthritis, but perhaps the main ones are:

— Rheumatoid arthritis
— Seronegative arthritis
— Gout
— Infections
— Malignancy
— Connective tissue disorders
— Osteoarthritis
— Inflammatory bowel disease.

It is clearly important to distinguish between the possibilities because the prognosis and the management of the different conditions are very different.

Questions for discussion

■ What questions might help you to suspect particular causes of polyarthritis and reject others?

■ Are there any clues in Mr Ibbotson's history to suggest what might be the cause of his arthritis?

■ Are there any features in Mr Ibbotson's history which might lead you to suspect a diagnosis of
  – lung cancer?
  – infection?
  – rheumatoid arthritis?

Activity 8.18

▶ Look again at the findings on physical examination in Mr Ibbotson. Clearly, he has a disorder that goes beyond the confines of a simple joint dysfunction.

▶ Refer back to Chapter 10 for more details on blood cell formation and to Chapter 1 for activities on percussing the chest.

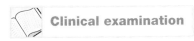

Clinical examination

▶ Look at the significance of a dullness to percussion combined with absent breath sounds. You will see that this combination of physical signs in the chest means that there is fluid in the pleural cavity.

Questions for discussion

■ What types of fluid may collect in the pleural cavity?

■ What is a pleural effusion?

■ Which causes of a pleural effusion might be relevant to Mr Ibbotson?

■ Which investigations would help you in determining the cause of a pleural effusion?

 Clinical examination

▶ Mr Ibbotson looks anaemic. Find out how you would test clinically for anaemia.

Questions for discussion

■ What is anaemia?

■ How reliable is physical examination in establishing the presence of anaemia?

■ How does the body compensate for the presence of anaemia?

■ How is anaemia classified?

■ What symptoms and signs may occur in an anaemic person, whatever the cause?

■ Which causes of anaemia do you think are relevant to Mr Ibbotson?

■ Which blood tests might help you determine the cause of Mr Ibbotson's anaemia?

 Medicine

▶ Look at how the pattern of joint involvement sometimes gives a clue as to the underlying cause. Note:

— The difference in which joints of the wrist and hand are affected in rheumatoid arthritis and osteoarthritis

— Which causes generally give rise to a symmetrical pattern of joint involvement

— The characteristics of joint swelling that can help you to distinguish between joint effusion, bony overgrowth and synovitis.

Questions for discussion

■ What type of joint swelling do you think Mr Ibbotson has?
■ Which causes of this type of joint swelling do you think are relevant to Mr Ibbotson?

Activity 8.19

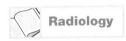 **Radiology**

▶ Look at a chest X-ray which shows a pleural effusion. (Refer back to Ch. 6 for another chest X-ray and Ch. 1 for more information on how to look at it.)
▶ Compare the two sides, and in particular the diaphragm shadows and the difference in the way which they dip laterally to form the costophrenic angle.

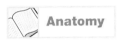 **Anatomy**

▶ Look at a textbook to see how the bases of the lower lung lobes dip down following the contour of the diaphragm.

The lowest part of the diaphragm in the erect or sitting person is located posteriorly, and pleural fluid will gravitate into this area. This means that a small pleural effusion may not be visible in the posteroanterior (PA) view but visible on the lateral view. As more fluid accumulates, it becomes visible on the PA view where it fills in the costophrenic angle on that side. With still more fluid present, the diaphragmatic shadow is obliterated and there is a U-shaped opacity on the X-ray.

Questions for discussion

■ What is a 'fluid level' in a pleural effusion?
■ Under what circumstances would you see a fluid level with a pleural effusion?

Activity 8.20

▶ Figure 8.1 is a plain X-ray of Mr Ibbotson's hands. Note the radiological anatomy of the bones of the wrist and hand and compare it with the anatomy of the bones from your study of them earlier in this case.

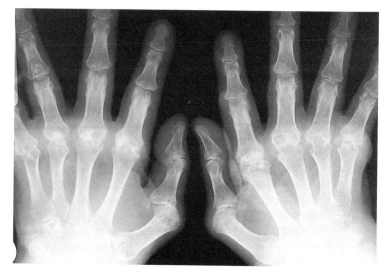

Fig. 8.1 A plain X-ray of Mr Ibbotson's hands.

▶ Compare Figure 8.1 with an X-ray of a normal hand. Note particularly the following features in Figure 8.1:
— An increase in soft tissue shadowing
— Narrowing of joint spaces
— Erosion of bone at the margins of joints.

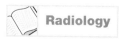 **Radiology**

▶ Find out if these features are found in particular forms of arthritis.

Question for discussion

■ In which other types of disorder may X-rays of the hand be useful?

Examination 2

Mr Ibbotson had a sample of blood taken from a vein in the antecubital fossa. The sample was tested in various ways. First, a full blood count was performed. The results were as follows:

Haemoglobin   11.5 g dl⁻¹
White cell count $9.0 \times 10^9 \, l^{-1}$

Platelet count	$280 \times 10^9 \, l^{-1}$
Mean corpuscular volume	80 fl
Mean corpuscular haemoglobin	30 pg
Mean corpuscular haemoglobin concentration	32 g dl^{-1}
Rheumatoid factor	1:40 dilution

Questions for discussion

- What type of anaemia does Mr Ibbotson have?
- What causes of this type of anaemia can you think of?
- Which further investigations might be useful for Mr Ibbotson?
- How is the test to detect rheumatoid factor carried out?
- Is Mr Ibbotson's test rheumatoid positive?

Activity 8.21

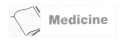 **Medicine**

▶ Study the causes of anaemia.

You will note from the above results that Mr Ibbotson has a mild anaemia and that the cells are of normal size (normocytic) and have a normal amount of haemoglobin in them (normochromic). Anaemia occurs if there is:

— Reduced production of red cells
— Increased destruction of red cells
— Loss of blood faster than the bone marrow can compensate.

Question for discussion

- Which of the causes of normocytic anaemia might be relevant in Mr Ibbotson's case, taking into account the history and physical examination, and the X-ray findings?

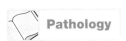 **Pathology**

▶ Another test measured the presence of rheumatoid factor in Mr Ibbotson's blood. Study the information that you have on rheumatoid factor. You will note that there are several rheumatoid factors, which are autoantibodies directed against the body's own immunoglobulin. The tests in general use measure IgM, although there are rheumatoid factors that belong to the IgG and IgA classes of immunoglobulin.

Questions for discussion

- What percentage of people with rheumatoid arthritis have a positive test for rheumatoid factor?
- What percentage of people with rheumatoid factor have rheumatoid arthritis?
- What other disorders may give rise to a positive rheumatoid factor test?

Examination 3

Mr Ibbotson had a test to drain some of the fluid from his chest. A sample of this was sent to the pathology laboratory for analysis. The results were as follows:

Appearance   Straw coloured, not turbid or bloodstained
Microscopy   No blood cells present
              No malignant cell present
Biochemistry Glucose content low
              Protein 4 g dl^{-1}
Culture   Sterile

Question for discussion

- Have the results of the analysis of pleural fluid altered your view of the cause of Mr Ibbotson's problems?

Activity 8.22

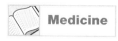 **Medicine**

▶ By this time, it should be reasonably clear that Mr Ibbotson has rheumatoid arthritis. Study the section in your textbook on rheumatoid arthritis.

You will have noted the involvement of the immune system in the production of the pathological features and the production of inflammatory mediators and enzymes which lead to characteristic destruction of bone and cartilage.

Note particularly the pattern of involvement of the joints and the associated systemic upset which may accompany a rapid onset of this condition.

From the point of view of Mr Ibbotson's case, the main point is that there are a number of extra-articular manifestations of rheumatoid arthritis which may affect up to 75% of patients. Note the wide variety of organs that may be affected, and also that sometimes the extra-articular manifestations may overshadow the joint problems.

Question for discussion

■ How may the muscles be affected in rheumatoid arthritis?

Activity 8.23

 Medicine

▶ Now look at the principles of management of a person with rheumatoid arthritis. Note the following aspects:

— Control of pain

— Prevention of disability

— Retaining function.

Drug therapy in rheumatoid arthritis, although important, is only a small part of the total management of the patient. Nevertheless, it is important to understand the principles of drug therapy, and in particular some of the important side-effects of the drugs.

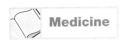 **Pharmacology / medicine**

▶ Study the drug treatment of rheumatoid arthritis. In particular note the pharmacology of the non-steroidal anti-inflammatory drugs (NSAIDs) such as aspirin and indomethacin. Study their action on the inflammatory process, and relate their pharmacology to some of their side-effects, particularly in the following areas:

— Stomach

— Kidneys

— Liver

— Nervous system

— Blood

— Skin

— Lungs.

Question for discussion

■ Do you think that Mr Ibbotson suffered any side-effects of NSAIDs?

The following drugs will be considered if treatment with anti-inflammatories does not reduce the inflammation after a few months:

— Sulphasalazine

— Chloroquine

— D-penicillamine

— Gold salts.

Question for discussion

■ Which side-effects of the drugs would be of relevance to a manual therapist?

▶ Now look at the use of corticosteroids in suppressing the inflammation of rheumatoid arthritis. They are powerful anti-inflammatory agents and also modify the immune response, but they have a number of potentially serious side-effects, particularly if they are used for a long time.

Questions for discussion

■ Which side-effects of corticosteroids might affect your management of a patient such as Mr Ibbotson?

■ How would you decide whether Mr Ibbotson was suitable for starting treatment with corticosteroids?

■ In which other conditions are corticosteroids used?

■ Do corticosteroids influence the ultimate course of rheumatoid arthritis?

■ By which routes may corticosteroids be given in rheumatoid arthritis?

In patients with severe rheumatoid arthritis who have not responded to the drugs mentioned earlier, immunosuppressive

agents such as methotrexate, azathioprine and
cyclophosphamide may be used.

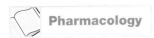
Pharmacology

▶ Study how these agents affect the immune response. Note
also their serious side-effects, particularly on the lungs and
liver, and the increased susceptibility to a wide range of
infectious agents.

Question for discussion

■ If, as a manual therapist, you had to treat a patient who was taking
immunosuppressive drugs, would you take any special precautions?

Although drugs can help with the control of pain and reduction
of inflammation, the progress of the disease may still mean that
there is much deformity, disability and loss of function. Manual
therapists can play a vital part in preventing such complications,
or at least in minimising their impact.

Questions for discussion

■ As a manual therapist what do you think the aim of your
management of Mr Ibbotson would be?

■ Which types of therapy would you use?

■ Are there any precautions that you would take with your therapy?

Activity 8.24

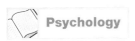
Psychology

▶ Finally, it is important not to forget the psychological impact
of Mr Ibbotson's illness. There are several issues to consider,
including:

— The anxiety and distress produced by the physical
symptoms

— The waiting for test results

— If the differential diagnosis included a potentially life-
threatening disease such as cancer, the feelings associated
with uncertainty over whether or not cancer is present

— The feelings produced when Mr Ibbotson is told that the disease is not life threatening but nevertheless incurable

— The feelings produced by the potential effect of the disease on Mr Ibbotson's work as a designer, and the financial and social implications of losing his job.

Questions for discussion

■ What factors might be important in determining Mr Ibbotson's ability to cope with the disease in the long term?

■ How would you help Mr Ibbotson cope with the psychological impact of his illness?

Discussion

This is a complex and interesting case. Mr Ibbotson has an acute onset of polyarthritis which affects both large and small joints, together with a general constitutional upset with weight loss and fever. In addition there are signs of anaemia and of a pleural effusion. There are no signs of cardiac failure (which would include all or some of cyanosis, raised jugular venous pressure, pitting oedema, enlarged liver, enlarged heart, tachycardia, third heart sound, and crepitations at the lung bases). The swellings in the fingers are almost certainly tendon sheath effusions.

There are many diseases that can cause a polyarthritis. The first question to answer is whether the arthritis is the primary disorder or whether it is part of another underlying condition. This may be very difficult to determine, particularly early on in the course of the illness, but it is important from the standpoint of patient management to try to reach as precise a diagnosis as possible quickly. The history and thorough physical examination is very important in this respect.

The main questions to ask the patient are related to the chronology (i.e. the onset and subsequent course of the condition), the pattern of joint involvement and the presence of any associated systemic symptoms such as fever, malaise and loss of weight. A hyperacute onset typically occurs in gout, where the joint becomes exquisitely painful over a period of a few minutes, but more frequently the progression is over a few weeks and involves a number of joints. This can occur with rheumatoid arthritis (RA) and other connective tissue disorders such as systemic lupus erythematosus (SLE). The pattern of joint involvement is important. For example, RA usually spares the distal interphalangeal joints of the hands while attacking the other joints, while psoriatic arthritis and osteoarthritis (OA) often attack the distal interphalangeal joints. SLE may be very difficult to distinguish from RA in the early stages. Peripheral arthritis occurs in about 20% of cases of ankylosing spondylitis, usually affecting proximal large joints such as hips and knees.

Systemic symptoms may occur in many connective tissue diseases and also in the arthritis which sometimes accompanies neoplastic disease. In a patient with a short history, it is important to exclude a local infective cause, but some systemic infections such as subacute bacterial endocarditis may give rise to an arthritis even though there is no direct joint invasion by organisms. RA is often associated with a number of so-called 'extra-articular manifestations', such as pleural effusion, pericarditis, peripheral neuropathy and an enlarged spleen; so are many connective tissue diseases, and of course malignancy may be associated with a general systemic upset as well as features of the primary tumour or its metastases.

In the case of Mr Ibbotson, the differential diagnosis is quite wide. The onset and pattern of involvement is consistent with RA and SLE; the lung problem would also support either of these diagnoses. The fact that he is a smoker raises the possibility of a lung cancer, a condition in which a pleural effusion is common. His recent holiday in Ireland might suggest that he has contracted tuberculosis (although the history is a little short) or has drunk milk infected with brucellosis. Subacute bacterial endocarditis often causes a cardiac murmur, but so does anaemia from any cause, and malignancy, RA, SLE and gastrointestinal blood loss from the anti-inflammatory drugs would all be good reasons for the anaemia.

Investigations should start with simple blood tests and radiology. A full blood count will confirm the anaemia and demonstrate its type. A high white cell count may occur to some extent in most inflammatory arthritides, but might indicate an infective cause. The ESR will probably be elevated whatever the cause. The blood should also be tested for rheumatoid factor and for antinuclear factor, and blood cultures taken. A chest X-ray will show the pleural effusion and may show signs of tuberculosis or lung cancer.

In the acute phase of an inflammatory arthritis, manipulation, articulation or soft tissue work are all contraindicated. When the inflammatory process is quiescent, it is possible to gently articulate the affected joints, give exercises and alter the diet to accommodate any food intolerances.

FURTHER READING

Bell M J, Bombardier C, Tugwell P 1990 Measurement of functional status, quality of life and utility in rheumatoid arthritis. Arthritis and Rheumatism 33: 591–601

Krol B, Sanderman R, Suurmeijer T, Doeglas D, van Rijswijk M, van
Leeuwen M 1995 Medical, physical and psychological status related
to early rheumatoid arthritis. Clinical Rheumatology 14: 143–150

Semble E L 1995 Rheumatoid arthritis: new approaches for its
evaluation and management. Archives of Physical Medicine and
Rehabilitation 76: 190–201

Case 9
Mr James Kirk

Study objectives

After studying this case with its associated activities and questions, you should have a reasonable knowledge of the following areas:

1. Surface anatomy of structures in the face and anterior part of the head
2. Anatomy of the bones of the face and anterior part of the skull, particularly the mandible, maxilla and temporal bone
3. Attachments, actions, blood and nerve supply of the muscles of facial expression
4. Attachments, actions, blood and nerve supply of the muscles of mastication
5. Course of the trigeminal nerve
6. Testing the motor and sensory functions of the trigeminal nerve
7. Course of the facial nerve
8. Testing the muscles of facial expression
9. Structure of the temporomandibular joint
10. Biomechanics of temporomandibular joint movement
11. Arterial supply to the face
12. Venous drainage of the face
13. Lymphatic drainage of the scalp
14. Relations of the parotid gland
15. Histology of the parotid gland
16. Factors influencing saliva production
17. Physiological mechanisms of saliva production
18. Concept of trigger points
19. Measurement of the erythrocyte sedimentation rate (ESR)
20. Significance of a raised ESR
21. Causes of pain in the face
22. Cellular events in the chronic inflammatory process

23. Differences between acute and chronic inflammation
24. Pathology of temporal arteritis
25. Clinical features of temporal arteritis
26. Complications of temporal arteritis
27. Treatment of temporal arteritis.

Background

James Kirk was fed up with Star Trek jokes, although he had just retired as Captain on a large liner which cruised all over the world. Being 65, and having a nice company pension, he was relishing the prospect of retirement, and did not want any tiresome symptoms to get in his way. So when he developed a headache, he expected you to give his neck 'a quick tweak' and that would get rid of it. However, despite his seeming impatience for you to get on with the job, you managed to persuade him that you always took the time to take a full history and perform a thorough physical examination. In retrospect, you felt glad that you did.

In fact, Mr Kirk admitted to quite a number of symptoms in the previous 6 months, but none of them seemed severe enough to warrant a visit to either you or his general practitioner. He thought they were just part of the ageing process and that he would be told that he would 'just have to live with it'. As far as the headache was concerned, it had been gradually increasing in severity over the past month or so, and was beginning to make him feel a little off-colour, so that his appetite was not as robust as it had been previously. The pain was located mainly in the left temple, but sometimes went to the jaw, especially when he was eating a piece of tough meat. Nothing in particular seemed to make it better or worse, but he had noticed that combing his hair produced quite a tender feeling in the area where his pain was located.

Questions for discussion

■ What are your initial thoughts about the cause of Mr Kirk's headache?

- Why might Mr Kirk experience jaw pain on eating?
- What other questions would you ask Mr Kirk?

The only other symptom that Mr Kirk admitted to was some stiffness across both shoulders which had been present for about 3 months. This was worse first thing in the morning and took about an hour to settle down. Mr Kirk had no drowsiness, nausea, vomiting or dizziness, nor had he experienced any tingling, numbness or weakness of the limbs. Systems review revealed no further symptoms, and in particular no toothache, visual disturbance or pain in the ear.

Questions for discussion

- Have you managed to narrow down your list of possible diagnoses?
- What would you particularly look for in the physical examination?

Pain in the face may arise from a wide variety of causes, and very often the patient may have no obvious abnormality on physical examination. This means that the history is of great importance in establishing a diagnosis.

A knowledge of the local anatomy and patterns of pain referral is clearly a crucial starting point in analysing this symptom. Face pain may arise from a number of structures, including:

— Eyes and orbit
— Teeth
— Paranasal sinuses
— Jaw
— Parotid gland
— Tongue
— Pharynx
— Blood vessels
— Nerves.

The main nerve supplying the face is the trigeminal nerve, although the glossopharyngeal and oculomotor nerves may cause pain in particular areas. As far as Mr Kirk is concerned, the pain is located mainly in the jaw and temporal region, and so for this case you will need to spend more time studying these areas.

Activity 9.1

▶ On your partner's head, identify the following structures by observation and by palpation:
  — Mastoid process
  — Zygomatic arch
  — Temporalis muscle
  — Masseter muscle
  — Sternocleidomastoid muscle
  — Parotid gland
  — Submandibular gland
  — Prominence of cheek
  — Nasion
  — Frontalis muscle
  — Temporal artery
  — Angle of jaw
  — External auditory meatus
  — Facial artery
  — Glabella
  — Supraorbital notch.

Activity 9.2

▶ Look at the skin of your partner's face. Examine the distribution of hair on it (females have some hair on the face, although it is usually much finer than in males). Note:
  — Any hairs on the nose
  — The thickness of the eyebrows, and whether there is any difference in hair density between the medial and lateral aspects of the eyebrow.
▶ Note whether your partner's face is moist from sweat or secretions from the sebaceous glands.
▶ Feel the texture of your partner's face. Are there areas where the skin is more firmly attached to the underlying structures? Gently lift a fold of skin from under the eyes, and compare its

thickness with a similar fold of skin from the cheek and from under the chin.

▶ Examine the colour of your partner's face. Are there areas of redness in the cheeks, or are they pale? Note any pigmentation, either in specific areas or of the whole face. (There is more information on the skin and fascia of the head in Ch. 5.)

Questions for discussion

■ Why are the lips pink?

■ What do you think is the mechanism of blushing?

■ What do you think is the mechanism of suntanning?

Activity 9.3

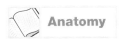 **Anatomy**

▶ Using your textbook, and relating the findings to your partner's head, note the position of the following structures:
  — Frontal bone
  — Nasal bone
  — Nasal cartilage
  — Zygomatic bone
  — Maxilla
  — Mandible
  — Parietal bone
  — Squamous part of temporal bone
  — Greater wing of sphenoid bone.

▶ Look at the following points on the skull:
  — Bregma
  — Lambda
  — Pterion.

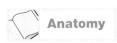 **Anatomy**

▶ Study some of the bones of the face in a little more detail. (It might be useful to have a model skull to hand while you are doing this, and you should note where the structures are on your partner's head.) First, identify the following parts of the mandible:

— Body

— Angle

— Ramus

— Condyle

— Coronoid process

— Mental foramen.

▶ Examine how the condyle of the mandible fits into the glenoid fossa of the temporal bone.

▶ Examine how the zygomatic bone connects with several of the bones of the face (which?).

▶ Note the maxilla forming the upper jaw and identify the following structures on it:

— Infraorbital foramen

— Anterior nasal spine

— Frontal process

— Zygomatic process

— Alveolar process.

▶ Look at how the maxilla extends backwards and forms part of the floor of the orbit. Note the temporal bone above the jaw and the temporomandibular joint just in front of the ear.

▶ Identify the following structures on the temporal bone:

— Mastoid process

— Styloid process

— Squama

— Middle ear.

Activity 9.4

▶ Ask your partner to:

— Puff out his cheeks

— Smile

— Bare his teeth

— Turn down the angles of his mouth

— Screw up his eyes

— Raise his eyebrows

— Pucker his lips

— Flare his nostrils.

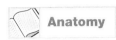 **Anatomy**

▶ Study the muscles of facial expression. Note the occipitofrontalis muscle, which covers the whole of the top of the skull. Note its actions in raising the eyebrows and wrinkling the forehead, giving the face an expression of surprise or even horror.

There are many other muscles of facial expression, and it is not necessary for you to know the Latin names of all of them. They are generally named in accordance with what they do (e.g. depressor septi) or where they are (e.g. nasalis). For example, the tongue-twister 'musculus levator labii superioris alaeque nasi' is a muscle which lifts the upper lip and the wing of the nose. Simple if you know your Latin! You do, however, need to be aware of the range of facial movements that the muscles can produce.

▶ When you are next talking with a group of people, notice (discreetly) the range of facial expressions that they display. Can you tell whether someone is anxious or depressed, angry or shy? Some people seem to have a permanent furrow in their brow. What do you think this signifies?

Questions for discussion

■ Which muscles are responsible for the movements that your partner performed earlier in this activity?

■ Which muscles of facial expression do you use when blowing a trumpet?

■ Which muscles of facial expression are active when you cry?

■ Can you think of other ways in which muscles can show our emotions?

■ What is a Bell's palsy and what disabilities does it produce?

Activity 9.5

▶ Ask your partner to:

— Clench his teeth

— Open his mouth

— Move his jaw backwards and forwards

— Move his jaw from side to side.

▶ Identify the masseter and temporalis muscles. Place your finger on your partner's masseter muscle as he repeatedly clenches and unclenches his teeth.

▶ Repeat this while palpating the temporalis muscle.

▶ Get a small piece of cotton wool and a pin, and gently touch the skin of your partner's face with each.

▶ Ask your partner to close his eyes and report whether the sensation he feels is 'sharp' or 'blunt', while you touch his face with either the cotton wool or the pin in a random sequence.

▶ Test three or four places in the following areas of the face on each side, noting whether your partner can consistently distinguish between sharp and blunt touch:

— Forehead

— Cheek

— Chin.

▶ Draw out a small piece of cotton wool into a wisp and gently touch it onto your partner's cornea, noting the reaction of your partner's eyes. (Do not do this more than once on each side, otherwise you may irritate the cornea.)

Questions for discussion

■ What is shingles?

■ What symptoms and signs would be produced if the ophthalmic division of the trigeminal nerve were affected by shingles?

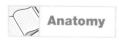 **Activity 9.6**

Anatomy

▶ Study the course of the trigeminal and facial nerves (see also the information on cranial nerves in Ch. 5). Note:

— That the trigeminal nerve has three divisions, and that the ophthalmic and maxillary divisions are entirely sensory whereas the mandibular division contains both sensory and motor nerve fibres

— The trigeminal ganglion in the petrous temporal bone; this is equivalent to a dorsal root ganglion in the spinal nerves.

▶ Trace the course of the ophthalmic division in the lateral wall of the cavernous sinus and note:

— Its division into frontal, lacrimal and nasociliary branches

— The area of sensory supply of each of the branches

— That the lacrimal nerve receives postganglionic parasympathetic nerve fibres from the pterygopalatine ganglion (the parasympathetic supply helps to regulate the production of tears).

▶ Trace the maxillary division as it passes through the foramen rotundum of the skull and divides into several branches to supply sensory fibres to the cheek and upper lip and the deep structures of the upper jaw.

▶ Note the position of the pterygopalatine ganglion, and study its neural connections.

▶ Trace the mandibular division.

The sensory root leaves the trigeminal ganglion while the motor root arises from cell bodies in the pontine region of the brain stem. The two roots join to pass through the foramen ovale in the skull and divide into a number of branches:

— Auriculotemporal nerve

— Lingual nerve

— Inferior alveolar nerve.

▶ Trace the course of each of these nerves and define their respective areas of sensory supply. Note the motor nerves supplying the muscles of mastication.

▶ Now trace the course of the facial nerve.

The facial nerve contains both sensory and motor nerve fibres; the motor fibres have their cell bodies in the pons, while those of the sensory fibres are in the geniculate ganglion in the petrous temporal bone. The course of the facial nerve is in close proximity to the vestibulocochlear nerve, from its exit from the pons, across the cerebellopontine angle and into the internal auditory meatus to reach the geniculate ganglion, and exit the skull via the stylomastoid foramen. Outside the skull, the facial nerve is entirely motor, and divides into several branches to supply the muscles of facial expression, including the buccinator and platysma. (See also Ch. 5.)

▶ Note:

— The chorda tympani, which carries both sensory and secretomotor fibres, as it passes into the infratemporal fossa just behind the temporomandibular joint

— The neural connections of the chorda tympani with the lingual nerve (define its area of sensory supply)

— The salivary glands which are supplied by the secretomotor fibres of the chorda tympani.

Activity 9.7

▶ Ask your partner to repeat the jaw movements of Activity 9.5. This time, palpate the movement of the temporomandibular joint (TMJ). Ask your partner to open his mouth as widely as possible while you do this. On some people it is possible to palpate a 'click' as the head of the mandible moves forwards in the mandibular (glenoid) fossa.

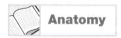 **Anatomy**

▶ Study the structure of the temporomandibular joint. Note:

— That it is a synovial joint

— The presence of a fibrocartilaginous disc which separates the head of the mandible from the mandibular fossa

— The joint is incongruous – i.e. the concavity of the mandibular fossa is different from the convexity of the condyle of the mandible

— The ovoid surface of the condyle, and the sellar (saddle-shaped) surface of the fossa, which constrains the movement of the joint to a gliding motion.

▶ Carefully palpate your partner's TMJ as he slowly opens his mouth, paying particular attention to the movement of the head of the mandible. In the first 30° or so of movement, the head of the mandible rotates, while after this it moves forward on the fossa.

▶ Study the details of TMJ movement, noting particularly:

— The deformation of the intra-articular disc

— The attachments of the disc to the joint capsule and condyle of the mandible

— The lateral pterygoid muscle and its attachment to the anterior part of the disc

— The attachments of the joint capsule.

▶ Note:

— The attachments of the various ligaments around the TMJ

— The temporomandibular ligament on the lateral side of the joint, and its attachments to the zygomatic bone and to the neck of the mandible

— The sphenomandibular ligament on the medial side of the joint and its attachments to the sphenoid bone and to the lingula of the mandibular foramen

— The stylomandibular ligament stretching from the styloid process to the ramus of the mandible.

Questions for discussion

■ What is the position of rest of the temporomandibular joint?

■ Do you think that Mr Kirk has arthritis of his temporomandibular joint?

■ In which direction can the mandible be dislocated?

■ What effects may be produced in the TMJ by abnormalities of the occlusal relationships of the teeth?

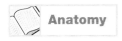 **Anatomy**

▶ Study the muscles that move the jaw. Note the attachments, actions, nerve supply and blood supply of the following muscles:

— Temporalis

— Masseter

— Lateral pterygoid

— Medial pterygoid

— Digastric

— Mylohyoid.

Questions for discussion

■ How are the muscles of mastication used in

– talking

- yawning
- chewing
- protrusion of the mandible
- retraction of the mandible?

■ Where are the trigger points for the masseter and temporalis muscles? What is the area of pain referral if one of these trigger points is activated?

■ Do you think that Mr Kirk has trigger point activity in his muscles of mastication?

▶ Ask your partner to relax his lower jaw so that his mouth is slightly open. Put your left index finger on your partner's lower jaw just below the lower lip. Now tap the finger sharply but not forcefully with a reflex hammer. You should find that the masseter and temporalis muscles contract and the jaw may close.

The jaw reflex is interesting because it is a monosynaptic reflex, but the central synaptic connection is in the pontine region of the brain rather than in the spinal cord.

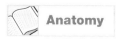

Anatomy

▶ Note the afferent and efferent limbs of the reflex in the mandibular division of the trigeminal nerve.

Activity 9.8

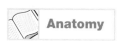

Anatomy

▶ In Activity 9.1 you should have been able to palpate the pulsation of the temporal and facial arteries. Now it is time to study the blood supply to the face. Note:

— The bifurcation of the common carotid artery at the upper border of the thyroid cartilage, and the course of the external carotid artery as it passes upwards into the parotid gland

— The division of the external carotid artery into the maxillary and superficial temporal arteries at the level of the neck of the mandible

— That many of the branches of the external carotid artery are looped in order to avoid stretching when the jaw, neck and pharynx are moved
— The course and distribution of the lingual artery as it supplies the floor of the mouth and the tongue
— The course of the facial artery as it curves upwards deep to the submandibular gland, emerging on the face just in front of the masseter muscle at the lower border of the mandible (it is palpable in this area)
— The branches of the facial artery, particularly to the pharynx, soft palate, tonsil, salivary glands, lip, nose and lacrimal sac
— The superficial temporal artery as it passes upwards from the parotid gland, giving branches to the temporomandibular joint, the ear, face and scalp
— The maxillary artery, which also begins in the parotid gland, passing into the infratemporal fossa and the pterygopalatine fossa
— Its branches, supplying the structures of
  – the ear
  – the meninges
  – the teeth and gums
  – the palate
  – the nose
  – the paranasal sinuses
  – the muscles of mastication
  – the temporomandibular joint.
▶ Note the extensive anastomoses between arteries in the face and scalp. The superficial temporal in particular has abundant anastomotic connections with:
— Its contralateral fellow
— The posterior auricular artery
— The occipital artery
— The supraorbital artery
— The supratrochlear artery.

Questions for discussion

■ Why does a wound to the scalp cause profuse bleeding?

■ If Mr Kirk had pain due to ischaemia of the muscles of mastication, which arteries might be involved?

Activity 9.9

▶ Ask your partner to perform a Valsalva manoeuvre. This involves trying to blow air out against a closed glottis, such as you might do if you were straining to pick up a heavy weight. Look at his face, and note whether the veins on the face become more prominent. Your partner's face may become reddened as the veins engorge with blood.

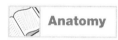 **Anatomy**

▶ Now consider the venous drainage of the face and scalp. Note in particular the extensive communication between intracranial and extracranial veins via the emissary veins. Note that there is great individual variation in the venous drainage.

▶ Study the course of the supratrochlear and supraorbital veins as they drain into the facial vein and communicate with the ophthalmic vein. Most of the face is drained by the facial vein which runs from the medial angle of the eye to the angle of the mandible. The occipital, superficial temporal and posterior auricular veins drain the rest of the scalp. Note how the veins draining the face join either the internal or external jugular veins, which then pass into the subclavian veins.

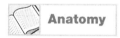 **Anatomy**

▶ Study the lymphatic drainage of the scalp. Note the superficial lymphatic vessels following the venous drainage and draining into groups of lymph nodes arranged around the base of the skull.

▶ Study in particular the following groups of lymph nodes, and the areas that they drain:
— Parotid
— Submandibular
— Submental
— Mastoid.

▶ Lymphatic vessels from these nodes drain into either the upper or lower deep cervical lymph nodes.

▶ While you are looking at the lymphatic drainage of the face, note the ring of lymphatic tissue around the oropharynx, commonly known as the tonsils and adenoids, which drain deep structures of the nose, orbit and pharynx and drain into the right and left cervical trunks.

Activity 9.10

▶ Collect the saliva produced by your partner over a timed period (about 10 minutes) and measure its volume.

▶ Ask your partner to chew on a piece of chewing gum and repeat the collection over the same amount of time. Unless your partner has a disorder which dries up salivary secretions, you should find that the volume has greatly increased after chewing the gum.

▶ Repeat the collection later on, when the taste has gone from the chewing gum. Ask your partner to think of a tasty meal, and determine whether this affects the rate of saliva production.

Questions for discussion

■ Have you ever had to speak in public and found that your mouth has dried up? Or have you had a surgical operation and found that the pre-med made your mouth dry? Discuss the reasons for these phenomena.

Activity 9.11

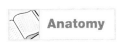 **Anatomy**

▶ Look at the position of the major salivary glands. For this case, because Mr Kirk had pain in the jaw, you should concentrate on the parotid gland. Note:
 — Its relationship to the masseter muscle, mastoid process, sternocleidomastoid muscle and ramus of the mandible
 — The deep cervical fascia enveloping the gland, and the branches of the facial nerve which pierce it
 — The division of the external carotid artery and the formation of the retromandibular vein within the gland

— The lymph drainage of the gland into the upper deep cervical nodes.

▶ Now look at the parotid duct as it lies on the masseter muscle and pierces buccinator to pass into the mouth. Note particularly the nerve supply to the parotid gland, derived from the glossopharyngeal nerve, trigeminal nerve and from the plexus of sympathetic nerves on the external carotid artery.

Questions for discussion

■ What symptoms do you think might be produced if the parotid duct were blocked by a stone?

■ To which structures would a surgeon operating on the parotid gland need to pay special attention?

Activity 9.12

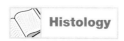 **Histology**

▶ Look at the structure of the parotid gland. It is a typical exocrine gland, with secretory cells arranged like segments of an orange to form an acinus, and ducts coming from the acini which join together to eventually form the parotid duct.

Question for discussion

■ What differences are there between mucus-secreting and serum-secreting cells in the salivary glands?

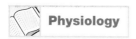 **Physiology**

▶ Now study the mechanism of salivary secretion.

The most important concept to grasp is that it is a two-stage process:

— The acini secrete a primary secretion, with mucin or ptyalin, and the concentration of ions in this is similar to that in the plasma

— The ducts modify the primary secretion by actively reabsorbing sodium and actively secreting potassium and bicarbonate ions.

The net result of this activity is that, under resting conditions, the sodium and chloride concentrations of saliva are low, whereas the potassium and bicarbonate concentrations are high.

Question for discussion

■ What differences are there in ionic composition between resting saliva and that collected during maximal salivation (such as with the chewing gum)? Account for these differences.

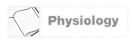

Physiology

▶ Look at the control of salivary secretion. The main stimulus comes from the parasympathetic nervous system, and is controlled by the salivary nuclei at the junction of the pons and medulla of the brain stem. Note the inputs to the salivary nuclei, partly from nerves arising from the mouth and tongue, but also from the areas of the brain responsible for sight, smell and thought, and also from the stomach and upper intestine.

▶ Note the outputs of the salivary nuclei to the facial and glossopharyngeal nerves, and to the cervical sympathetic ganglia.

Question for discussion

■ What differences are there between saliva produced by parasympathetic stimulation and that produced by sympathetic stimulation?

The blood flow to the salivary glands is an important factor in salivary secretion. During salivation, the activated cells produce kallikrein, which is converted to the powerful vasodilator bradykinin. This mechanism ensures that blood flow is increased when it is needed.

Questions for discussion

■ What functions of saliva can you think of?

■ Can you think of some disorders which will cause a reduction in the production of saliva?

■ What problems might be experienced by a person with reduced saliva production?

■ Do you think that Mr Kirk has a problem with his parotid gland?

Examination 1

On examination, Mr Kirk looked in reasonably good shape. He was well nourished and there was no evidence of anaemia or muscle wasting. Pulse, blood pressure and temperature were normal. Cardiovascular, respiratory and neurological examinations were entirely normal, as was abdominal palpation. There was quite a lot of tenderness in both trapezius muscles, with several trigger points referring pain to the occipital area and the jaw. There was another tender area in the left temple, at the site of the pain that Mr Kirk had described, and you had the impression that the left temporal artery was not pulsating as well as that on the right.

Questions for discussion

- Do the examination findings help you in forming your differential diagnosis?
- Are there any special investigations that you think might be helpful?
- Are there any special dangers associated with one of the diagnoses that should be on your list?
- How would you manage Mr Kirk?

The next activity is designed to help you think a little more deeply about trigger points. These arise in virtually every chapter in this book, and it is extremely important for you to be familiar with the concept of trigger points.

Activity 9.13

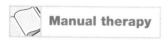 **Manual therapy**

▶ If you have a textbook which shows the trigger points for the various muscles, choose the one for the masseter muscle. Otherwise, locate the temporomandibular joint in your partner; the trigger point for the masseter is just anterior to this.

▶ Have your partner sitting with his back to you and press firmly with your right thumb into the point, and determine whether your partner finds it painful. Of course, if you press hard enough, it will be painful, but with a true active trigger point you will find that the pain is referred to a distant region. You may also find twitching or fasciculation of the muscle.

 Manual therapy

▶ Study the nature and origin of trigger points.

Trigger points are associated with localised muscle tenderness and hardening, and with referral of pain to a distant area. The precise neurophysiology of the genesis of trigger points is not known, but seems to involve hyperactivity of the spindles in the affected muscles. (There is further information on muscle spindles and their role in reflex activity in Ch. 4.) Note that there appears to be a lack of oxygen in the muscle at the location of a trigger point.

Questions for discussion

■ What differences do you think there are between trigger points and acupuncture points?

■ What factors can you think of that might enhance or perpetuate the activity of trigger points?

■ What methods are there for deactivation of trigger points?

■ How may 'satellite' trigger points originate?

■ What is fibromyalgia?

■ What differences do you think there are between fibromyalgia and multiple trigger points?

Examination 2

Mr Kirk had a blood test, which showed a normal full blood count, normal urea and electrolytes and normal liver function. However, the erythrocyte sedimentation rate (ESR) was substantially raised at 70 mm in the first hour. Chest X-ray showed no evidence of cancer or tuberculosis, and skull X-ray showed no evidence of raised intracranial pressure or of infiltration with tumour.

Questions for discussion

- What does the ESR measure? What is its normal value?
- What causes of a raised ESR can you think of?
- What features of a skull X-ray would suggest raised intracranial pressure?
- What are the clinical features of raised intracranial pressure?
- Do you think that Mr Kirk has raised intracranial pressure?
- What other investigations might be helpful in Mr Kirk?

Activity 9.14

▶ Collect together the materials you will need for this activity: a test tube or length of narrow glass tubing; a strong magnet; some magnetic material such as iron filings or a paper clip; some water; some viscous liquid such as vegetable oil or runny honey; and a plastic object such as a comb.

▶ First, put the water in the tube and put the iron filings on top of the liquid. They should fall rapidly to the bottom of the tube.

▶ Replace the water with a more viscous liquid and repeat the procedure. The filings will now fall more slowly through the liquid. Note the time taken for the filings to fall a certain distance, say 10 cm.

▶ Now repeat the experiment using the oil, but this time put the magnet under the tube (see Fig. 9.1). Note the time taken for the filings to fall 10 cm through the oil. You should find that the time is less with the magnet. You should also find that as the filings get closer to the magnet, the speed of fall increases (a phenomenon known as the 'inverse square law').

▶ Repeat all three experiments with a larger magnetic object such as a paper clip or panel pin. You should find that this falls more quickly through the liquids under all three conditions.

▶ Take the plastic comb and rub it vigorously against your sleeve. Now put the comb near to your hair. The hair should stand up as it is attracted towards the comb. This doesn't always work, particularly on a damp day, but I am sure that you have experienced examples of static electricity many times; for example when taking off your clothes (especially if they are made of nylon) you often hear a 'crackling' sound and the material clings to your skin.

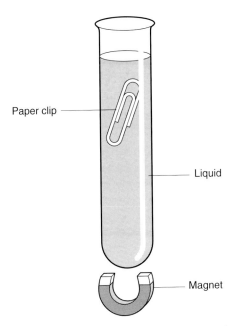

Fig. 9.1 Check the speed of fall of the paper clip as it approaches the magnet.

Question for discussion

■ What is the role of electrical charge in the phenomenon known as 'static electricity'?

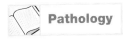 **Pathology**

▶ Study how the ESR is taken, and what its significance is.

The actual equipment used to measure the ESR is very simple (some blood-taking equipment, anticoagulant and a tube about 15 cm long). The tube is filled with the anticoagulated blood and stood vertically for 1 hour. After that time, the tube is inspected. The red blood cells will have packed down to a certain extent. The ESR is the distance in millimetres from the top of the column of blood to the top of the column of red cells (Fig. 9.2).

▶ Study the reasons why the red cells pack down.

The easiest one to understand is the difference in specific gravity between the red cells and the plasma. However, one of the most important pathological factors is the formation of red cell clumps (rouleaux). This happens when the red cells are attracted to each

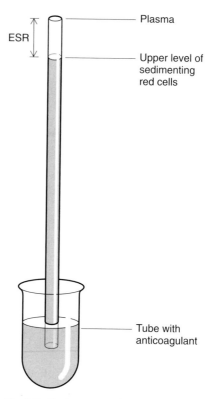

Fig. 9.2 Equipment used to measure ESR.

other by molecular charge, and this in turn occurs when there is an increase in the concentration of fibrinogen and certain globulins in the plasma.

Examination 3

Mr Kirk had a biopsy of his left temporal artery. It showed disruption of the internal elastic lamina, with a mononuclear cell infiltrate and multinucleated giant cells.

Questions for discussion

■ What is the diagnosis?
■ What would be your management of Mr Kirk?

Activity 9.15

▶ Study the characteristics of chronic inflammation (see also the activities regarding the inflammatory response in Ch. 8).

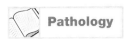 **Pathology**

▶ Study the differences between acute and chronic inflammation, noting in particular the cellular predominance of the chronic inflammatory process. Chronic inflammation may occur:

— As a result of unresolved acute inflammation

— As a chronic process right from the start.

▶ Note the types of cells which are present in a focus of chronic inflammation, particularly:

— Lymphocytes

— Fibroblasts

— Macrophages

— Plasma cells.

▶ There are many causes of chronic inflammation, and a similar histological picture may be produced. Note the different types of the chronic inflammatory response:

— Serous

— Fibrous

— Suppurative

— Ulcerative

— Granulomatous.

Questions for discussion

■ Do you see the cardinal features of inflammation (see Ch. 8 for definition) with the chronic inflammatory process?

■ What is granulomatous inflammation?

■ What are giant cells, and what factors cause their formation?

■ Do you think that Mr Kirk has a chronic inflammatory process going on?

Discussion

In the case of Mr Kirk, there are no features that might suggest an expanding intracranial lesion, nor are there any suggestions of infection, although his world-wide travel may have brought him into contact with all sorts of tropical diseases, including tuberculosis. There is no history of previous migraine, and although it can present for the first time in later life, often in association with hypertension, it is not common. 'Tension' headaches might be a possibility in Mr Kirk, since he has recently retired and might be anxious about what the future holds, despite his assertions that he is confident. The stiffness and trigger points across the shoulders might also support this. In people of Mr Kirk's age, cancer of any site metastasising to the brain must be well up on the list of diagnoses. Sometimes, symptoms associated with metastases occur before the manifestation of the tumour in the primary site, and anorexia, general malaise and loss of weight may be the only clues that a pathological process may be present.

Temporal (cranial) arteritis also occurs predominantly in people over the age of 60, and is a distinct possibility here. The headache of temporal arteritis may be of a non-specific tension character, or may be localised and associated with scalp tenderness. Pain in the jaw on chewing is due to facial artery claudication (see Ch. 3 for further discussion of vascular obstruction) and there may be tingling of the tongue and loss of taste for similar reasons. About half of sufferers have features of polymyalgia rheumatica, with proximal limb girdle pain, stiffness and tenderness, worse after rest. Often there are systemic symptoms of variable severity. Examination may reveal loss of temporal artery pulsation and localised muscle tenderness but often there is not much to find. The great danger with temporal arteritis is sudden, irreversible blindness, which is only sometimes preceded by visual disturbances. If this diagnosis is suspected, some authorities say that steroids should be started immediately to prevent visual complications while investigations are proceeding.

Investigation in Mr Kirk should include a full blood count and ESR to give a clue as to the presence of anaemia or leukaemia, or a general inflammatory process. Chest X-ray will show whether or not there is lung cancer while skull X-ray may show signs of raised intracranial pressure. Temporal artery biopsy will show if the changes of temporal arteritis are present. If there was any doubt as to whether there was a chronic inflammatory process causing the headaches, then a lumbar puncture should be performed.

As far as the manual therapist is concerned, it is important for the pathological process to be arrested before attempting any physical treatment. The trigger points may be treated appropriately, as may any restrictions in the upper cervical region of the spine. Restrictions in the temporomandibular joint may also be addressed.

The diagnosis in Mr Kirk was temporal arteritis, and he was started on 80 mg of prednisolone daily. His symptoms resolved after 2 days on this, and he remained well on follow-up at 6 months.

FURTHER READING

Caselli R J, Hunder G G 1993 Neurologic aspects of giant cell (temporal) arteritis. Rheumatic Disease Clinics of North America 19: 941–953

Lee A G 1995 A case report. Jaw claudication: a sign of giant cell arteritis. Journal of the American Dental Association 126: 1028–1029

Lie J T 1994 When is arteritis of the temporal arteries not temporal arteritis? Journal of Rheumatology 21: 186–189

Case 10
Mrs Christine Evans

After studying this case with its associated activities and questions, you should have a reasonable knowledge of the following areas:

1. Surface anatomy of structures on the posterior part of the thorax
2. Surface markings of the heart and lungs
3. General characteristics of a vertebra
4. Particular characteristics of the thoracic vertebrae
5. Attachments and functions of the ligaments of the thoracic vertebral column and ribs
6. Attachments, actions, blood and nerve supply of muscles of the posterior chest wall
7. Biomechanics of movements of the thoracic spine and thoracic cage
8. Testing movements of the thoracic spine as a whole
9. Testing movements between individual thoracic vertebrae
10. Formation of nerve roots from the spinal cord
11. Components of spinal nerves
12. Nerve supply to the posterior thorax
13. Histology of bone marrow
14. Formation of the cellular elements of the blood
15. Causes of anaemia
16. Clinical effects of anaemia
17. Examination of the abdomen
18. Features of enlargement of the various abdominal organs
19. X-ray appearances of the thoracic vertebrae
20. Separation of blood constituents by electrophoresis
21. Structure of paraproteins
22. Significance of the presence of a paraprotein in the blood

23. Histological appearances of malignant plasma cells
24. Differential diagnosis of pain in the posterior thorax
25. Clinical features of multiple myeloma
26. Principles of use of cytotoxic drugs
27. Side-effects of cytotoxic chemotherapy of relevance to manual therapists.

Background

It is a widely accepted belief in manual therapy practice that difficult cases usually arrive on a Saturday evening, when thoughts are beginning to turn to the prospect of tomorrow's fishing. There is little evidence to support this belief, but when Mrs Evans arrives with a long referral letter from her general practitioner, you are not surprised.

In the letter, the general practitioner told you that Mrs Evans was a 58-year-old cleaner, was married with three healthy children, smoked 30–40 cigarettes a day, and had many complaints. She had enjoyed reasonably good health until she suffered a pulmonary embolus about 18 months previously. Approximately 3 months after the embolus, when her dose of warfarin was being reduced, her symptoms began. Firstly, there was pain which seemed to travel from site to site. The most common site for the pain was between the shoulder blades, but she also complained of pain near the left sacroiliac joint, in the lumbar spine, and in the back of the neck. Second, there was a burning sensation which began in the feet and was gradually working its way upwards. Similar sensations were occurring in the fingertips. The general practitioner was wondering whether you 'might be able to do some work on her back to make her more comfortable'.

Question for discussion

■ What further history would you like to take from Mrs Evans?

On further questioning, there was a great deal more that Mrs Evans wanted to tell you. She had lost approximately 5 kg in weight over the previous 3 months and was feeling

increasingly weak. In particular, she was finding it difficult
to walk up the stairs to her bedroom and she felt that her
grip while polishing was not as good as it had been. She
was also finding that she was getting 'a bit out of puff'
during her work, a thing that she had never experienced
before. Another problem that she had noticed was that she
was having to go to the lavatory more frequently to pass
urine and was having to drink more 'to make up for losing
all that water'. The urine had also recently become a little
frothy. Despite this increase in her urinary frequency, she
felt that her bowel motions were rather sluggish, and she
experienced some abdominal cramping sensations when
she felt the desire to defaecate.

Question for discussion

■ You are probably getting quite confused by this plethora of
symptoms! Nevertheless, you have to perform some
examination. On which areas would you concentrate your
efforts?

Patients who have multiple symptoms can be very
challenging for the practitioner to deal with, and it can be
very difficult to know where to start. Many patients turn
out to have nothing seriously wrong with their physical
condition, but the physical symptoms may be a
manifestation of an underlying emotional conflict.
However, it would be quite wrong to assume that this is the
case before making a thorough attempt to elucidate a
potentially serious physical problem. Since Mrs Evans
experiences most of her pain in the thoracic region of the
spine, for this case you will concentrate on this for much of
your study.

Activity 10.1

▶ You will need your partner to strip to the waist for this
activity. On the back of your partner's chest, identify the
following structures:
— Spine of 1st thoracic vertebra
— Spine of 4th thoracic vertebra

— Superior angle of scapula
— Spine of scapula
— Inferior angle of scapula
— Spine of 8th thoracic vertebra
— Spine of 12th thoracic vertebra
— Posterior axillary fold
— Tendon of latissimus dorsi
— 12th rib.

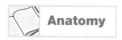

Anatomy

▶ Look at the surface markings of the lungs on the posterior chest wall.

▶ On your partner, mark the upper and lower limits of the lungs and pleura, and the oblique fissure of the right and left lungs.

▶ Use the technique of percussion (see Ch. 1), to delineate the extent of the lungs posteriorly. You may be surprised at how far down the lungs extend.

▶ Feel the ribs of your partner as they pass from their articulation with the vertebrae posteriorly around the chest wall.

▶ Ask your partner to take some deep breaths and note the motion of the ribs.

▶ Repeat this exercise for the upper, middle and lower ribs. Can you detect any differences? (There are further activities concerning the motion of the ribs in respiration in Ch. 1.)

Activity 10.2

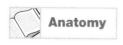

Anatomy

▶ If you have access to a set of disarticulated bones, take the 12 thoracic vertebrae for this activity. Otherwise, look in your textbook. Note:

— The general characteristics of a vertebra, in particular the body and the arch

— The roughened upper and lower surfaces of the body, for the attachment of the intervertebral discs

— The side-to-side convexity of the anterior surface and the slight concavity of the posterior surface
— The presence of the pedicles and laminae, and the spinous, articular and transverse processes
— The vertebral notches above and below the pedicles
— Note particularly that when two vertebrae are articulated with each other, the concavities of the vertebral notches of contiguous vertebrae form the intervertebral foramina.

Questions for discussion

■ What structures pass through the intervertebral foramen?
■ What functions does the vertebral column as a whole subserve?
■ Why do you think the vertebral column is made up of so many individual bones?

▶ Now study the thoracic vertebrae in a little more detail. Note:
— The gradual increase in size between the 1st and 12th thoracic vertebrae
— That the laminae are fairly small, and that the vertebral foramen (be careful to distinguish the vertebral foramen from the intervertebral foramen) is small and round.

▶ Look at the downward slope of the spinous processes, and note that in an articulated spine they overlap. This means that the palpable portion of the spinous process may not be in the same plane as the body of the same vertebra. Note in particular the costal facets on the sides of the bodies and on the transverse processes. These are for articulation with the heads and tubercles respectively of the ribs. You will see that there are two facets on the bodies of most of the thoracic vertebrae, but that the 9th to 12th usually have only one facet, implying that they articulate with only one rib.

▶ Look at the direction of the superior and inferior articular processes and their articular facets, which are oval in shape and flat or slightly convex transversely. Note the difference in direction of the inferior articular processes of T12.

Questions for discussion

■ Which movements between adjacent thoracic vertebrae do you think are facilitated and which may be restricted by the arrangement of the articular processes?

■ Discuss the concept that the thoracic part of the spine is merely a transitional zone between the cervical and lumbar spinal regions.

Activity 10.3

▶ Again, you will need your partner stripped to the waist. Have your partner seated so that you can stand behind him and manoeuvre his spine. Firstly, observe his back. Is there any obvious asymmetry or scoliosis?

▶ Look at the levels of the inferior angles of the scapulae; are they at the same horizontal level? Is one scapula more prominent?

▶ Run your index finger down the spine from T1 to T12, noting:
— Any deviation of a spinous process from the midline
— Any prominence of an individual spinous process
— Any tenderness of an individual spinous process (you will need to press a little more firmly on each spinous process to determine this feature).

▶ Using gentle pressure, slide the pads of your fingers over the transverse processes of T1 towards T12. Note whether there are any differences in the skin in terms of:
— Tenderness
— Firmness
— Moisture.

▶ Place your hands on your partner's shoulders so that the web space between the thumb and 1st finger on each hand is over the acromion; the thumb should rest gently on the posterior chest wall, pointing downwards towards T12, while the fingers rest on the anterior chest wall.

▶ Now push down gently but firmly in the direction of your thumbs with your right hand on your partner's right shoulder. His thoracic spine should bend to the right side (this is termed side-bending or lateral flexion). You might find it helpful to place the thumb or thenar eminence of your left hand on the right side of the spine of the 12th thoracic vertebra in order to fix the fulcrum of the movement.

▶ Repeat the exercise on the left side, and compare:
— The degree of lateral flexion to each side
— The smoothness of the vertebral curve produced
— The ease with which the lateral flexion is induced.

▶ Now repeat these manoeuvres with:

— Your hands so that they are halfway between the acromion and the neck, with the thumbs pointing towards T8

— Your hands placed as close as possible to your partner's neck with the thumbs pointing towards T4.

▶ In each case, note whether there is any asymmetry.

These manoeuvres test the motion of the thoracic spine between T1 and the thoracic vertebra to which the thumb is pointing. You should find that you need more pressure to move the spine as you move your hand towards your partner's neck.

Questions for discussion

■ What might be the significance of excessive tenderness to palpation at a particular level or levels in the thoracic spine?

■ How does the range of motion in the thoracic spine compare with that in the lumbar spine? What factors do you think influence any differences?

Activity 10.4

▶ This activity is broadly similar to the previous one, but this time you are going to test for motion between individual segments of the thoracic spine. There are many techniques for doing this, and you should not necessarily think that the activity you are going to perform now is the most appropriate for your particular discipline. Again, your partner should be stripped to the waist and seated with his back to you.

▶ Firstly, ask your partner to slump forwards, then rotate his trunk. Note the range of rotation to left and right.

▶ Ask him to sit up straight and repeat the rotation. You should find that the range of rotation is increased.

Question for discussion

■ Why should the range of rotation be greater when your partner is sitting up straight?

▶ Place your left hand on top of your partner's head. Place your right hand so that the 1st and 2nd fingers are extended and facing horizontally to the right, with the pad of the 1st finger resting on the spine of your partner's 1st thoracic vertebra and the pad of the 2nd finger resting on the spine of his 2nd thoracic vertebra. Now gently bend your partner's head forwards until you can detect motion of your fingers. You will need to concentrate quite hard when you are doing this, particularly if you have not done this before, since the range of motion is small and it is easy to bend your partner's head too far forwards.

▶ When your partner's head is bent forwards just enough for you to detect a separation of the spinous processes of T1 and T2, perform the following manoeuvres:

— Rotate your partner's head to the left and to the right until the spinous process of T1 starts to move relative to that of T2

— Side-bend your partner's head to the left and to the right again until the T1 spinous process moves relative to that of T2.

▶ Repeat these manoeuvres at successive levels down the thoracic spine. You will find that once you progress below about T4/5, you will need to induce motion in your partner's thoracic spine by reaching your left hand across the front of his chest and grasping his right shoulder. With a little practice, you will find that you can induce flexion, extension, side-bending and rotation quite easily. (Techniques similar to these are often used to mobilise the thoracic spine in a patient with restriction if the movements are repeated smoothly and rhythmically.) In each case try to compare the symmetry of movement.

Question for discussion

■ If your partner had a restriction of flexion and of side-bending and rotation to the right side at a particular level, how would you interpret this in terms of the movements of the thoracic vertebrae?

Activity 10.5

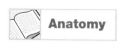 **Anatomy**

▶ Look at the ligaments of the thoracic vertebral column. Note the following:

— Anterior longitudinal ligament

— Posterior longitudinal ligament

— Supraspinous ligament
— Interspinous ligaments
— Intertransverse ligaments
— Ligamenta flava.

▶ Note also the presence of the intervertebral discs between the bodies of adjacent vertebrae (see also Chs 4 and 14).

▶ Study the ligaments of the joints between the vertebrae and the ribs. Note the fibrous capsules of the costovertebral and the costotransverse joints, and also the following:

— Radiate ligament
— Intra-articular ligament
— Costotransverse ligament
— Superior costotransverse ligament
— Lateral costotransverse ligament.

 Functional anatomy / biomechanics

▶ Study the movements of the thoracic spine. Note that the thoracic spine is capable of flexion, extension, lateral flexion and rotation.

During extension, the inferior articular process of the superior vertebra moves posteriorly and inferiorly on the superior articular process of the inferior vertebra, whereas in lateral flexion the articular surfaces on each side of a vertebra move in different directions, one moving up and the other moving down. During rotation, the articular facets on one vertebra move sideways relative to those on the adjacent vertebra.

▶ Put the different directions of motion in ascending order of movement.

Questions for discussion

■ Which structures limit movements in the various directions in the thoracic spine?

■ Lateral flexion of the thoracic vertebrae to one side is accompanied by rotation to the opposite side. Why do you think that this should be so?

■ Where is the axis of rotation in the thoracic vertebrae?

■ What differences do you think there are between rotation in the thoracic spine and in the lumbar spine?

Note in particular that the thoracic cage, consisting of the ribs, sternum and costal cartilages, has a major influence on the movement of the thoracic column as a whole. In general, the thoracic cage limits the movements which would be seen in the individual vertebrae, by stabilising the thoracic spine at the costovertebral and costotransverse joints and by increasing the inertia of the thoracic spine as a whole. This latter affect arises from an increase in the anteroposterior and transverse diameters of the thorax. Despite the fact that the individual components of the ribcage are fairly flexible, the presence of the ribcage substantially increases the stiffness of the thoracic column during its movements.

Questions for discussion

■ What happens during right lateral flexion to
  - the left intercostal spaces
  - the thoracic cage on the left side
  - the costochondral angle of the left 10th rib?
■ What happens to the ribs during rotation of the thoracic spine?

Activity 10.6

▶ Have your partner, stripped to the waist, sitting with his back to you and his feet about 20 cm apart on the floor. Ask him to lace his hands behind his neck and put his elbows forwards so that they are nearly touching in front of his head. Now have him bend forwards until his head is between his knees. Note the movement of the spine as a whole, and note particularly the contribution of the thoracic spine to the total range.

▶ Repeat the observations with your partner:
  — Arching his back to extend the spine as far as possible
  — Bending to each side
  — Rotating to each side.

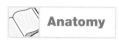 **Anatomy**

▶ Now study the muscles that produce these movements. Look at the layers of muscles on the posterior aspect of the trunk.

▶ Look at the paravertebral muscles attached directly to the vertebrae, and note particularly that the deeper the muscle is situated, the shorter it is.

▶ Look at the attachments, nerve supply and actions of the following muscles in the thoracic region:

— Iliocostalis

— Longissimus

— Spinalis

— Transversospinalis

— Rotatores

— Intertransversarii

— Serratus posterior inferior

— Latissimus dorsi.

These muscles generally act to extend the trunk, and when the sacrum is fixed the thoracolumbar joint is extended. Some of them also act as accessory muscles of respiration. However, the main function of the short muscles appears to be in posture, controlling the movements of adjoining vertebrae and preventing buckling of the spine while the long muscles actually perform the movements.

Activity 10.7

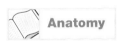 **Anatomy**

▶ Study the nerve supply to the thoracic region, and in particular consider whether individual tissues are capable of becoming the site of pain impulses. Note:

— How a spinal nerve is formed in the thoracic region

— The ventral and dorsal roots emerging from the spinal cord, the dorsal root ganglion and the arrangement of the coverings of the nerves (pia, arachnoid and dura)

— That the roots of the thoracic nerves are small relative to those in the cervical and lumbar regions.

Question for discussion

■ Why do you think that the thoracic nerve roots are relatively small?

▶ Look at the union of the dorsal and ventral roots to form the spinal nerve, and note the relationship of the spinal nerve to the intervertebral foramen.

▶ Study, in particular, the anatomy of the recurrent meningeal nerve.

The recurrent meningeal nerve is a sensory nerve which also contains fibres from the sympathetic ganglia. It arises from the spinal nerve and then re-enters the vertebral canal via the intervertebral foramen. It supplies the anterior and posterior longitudinal ligaments, the dura of the nerve roots, the blood vessels of the spinal cord and its membranes, and possibly the outer layer of the annulus fibrosus of the intervertebral disc. The recurrent meningeal nerve is believed to be the major sensory nerve of the vertebral functional unit.

▶ For each of the following tissue sites, determine whether it is capable of being a site of pain, and if it is, describe its nerve supply:
  — Intervertebral disc
  — Vertebral body
  — Facet joints
  — Anterior longitudinal ligament
  — Posterior longitudinal ligament
  — Other ligaments of the spine and ribs (see Activity 10.5)
  — Pia mater
  — Arachnoid mater
  — Dura mater
  — Spinal arteries
  — Spinal veins
  — Muscles on the back of the thorax
  — Tendons of the thoracic muscles
  — Dorsal root ganglion.

Question for discussion

■ What symptoms does irritation of a nerve root (from trauma, traction or pressure) produce?

The spinal nerve divides into dorsal and ventral rami (also termed posterior and anterior primary rami) just after the emergence of the recurrent meningeal nerve. The upper 11 of the ventral rami of the thoracic nerves lie between the ribs, whereas the 12th lies below the last rib and is called the subcostal nerve. The upper two thoracic nerves send branches to the brachial plexus, but the others are distributed mainly to the walls of the thorax and abdomen. Note that many diseases that affect the nerve trunks near their origins may give rise to chest or abdominal pain.

The dorsal ramus of each thoracic nerve passes backwards close to the facet joints and divides into medial and lateral branches.

▶ Follow the medial branch as it travels between the facet joint and the intertransverse muscle, and the lateral branch running laterally in the space between the superior costotransverse ligament and the intertransverse muscle, and then turning backwards medial to the levator costae muscle.

Question for discussion

■ Which structures are supplied by the medial and lateral branches of the dorsal rami of the thoracic nerves?

▶ Study the components of the spinal nerves. Each nerve contains fibres belonging to both somatic and visceral systems. Fibres from each system may be either afferent or efferent.

Question for discussion

■ Which structures in the thorax are supplied by the following types of nerve fibre
  - somatic afferent
  - somatic efferent
  - visceral afferent
  - visceral efferent?

Activity 10.8

▶ Go to your local butcher's shop and get some bones, preferably long bones, for example a leg of lamb would do nicely. (If you are not a vegetarian you may want to combine this activity with a meal.) There is further information about the structure of bones in Chapter 14, but for the purposes of this activity you should study the cavity of the bone. In a leg bone from a butcher's shop you may find some soft, pulpy material that can be scraped out from the central cavity. This is the bone marrow.

Questions for discussion

- What differences are there between red marrow and yellow marrow?
- Describe the changes that occur in the composition and distribution of the bone marrow with age.

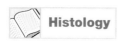 **Histology**

▶ Study the structure of bone marrow. Note:
— That the yellow marrow consists mainly of connective tissue and fat cells, whereas the red marrow has a framework of reticular connective tissue in which lie numerous blood cells of varying degrees of maturity
— The blood supply to the bone marrow from the nutrient artery which terminates in an extensive network of sinusoids
— The venous drainage, in which the sinusoids drain into large veins
— Note particularly the fact that the walls of the sinusoids are leaky, so that the maturing blood cells can enter the circulation when they reach maturity.

▶ Look at the formation of the cellular elements of the blood (haemopoiesis). It is believed that all the blood cells arise from a single type of cell (stem cell) which has the capability to differentiate into any of the different cell types. As the cell matures, this ability becomes restricted, and so the cell becomes committed to forming one type of cell.

Questions for discussion

- What are haemopoietic growth factors? Where are they produced and what are their functions?
- How does the body normally regulate the production of the different blood cell types?

■ What are the functions of

- – erythrocytes
- – neutrophils
- – eosinophils
- – basophils
- – monocytes
- – lymphocytes
- – platelets?

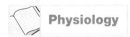 **Physiology**

▶ Study the stages of differentiation of the various blood cell types. For the moment, you should concentrate on the erythrocytes. Note:

— That the cells become smaller as they mature

— The change in staining properties as the cell fills with haemoglobin, and the loss of the nucleus in the later stages of maturation.

▶ Look at the regulation of erythrocyte production and the requirement for vitamin B_{12}, folic acid and iron. Note particularly the role of erythropoietin from the kidney in the stimulation of erythrocyte production, and the role of tissue oxygenation in the regulation of erythropoietin production.

Questions for discussion

■ What is 'anaemia'?

■ What is 'polycythaemia'? What is the difference between primary and secondary polycythaemia?

■ What factors can you think of that would decrease tissue oxygenation and so stimulate erythropoietin production?

■ What diseases might reduce the availability of vitamin B_{12} and folic acid to the developing erythrocytes?

■ What diseases might reduce the availability of iron to the developing erythrocytes?

▶ Study the development of the white cell series, in particular the two major lineages of white cells, namely the myelocytic and the lymphocytic. Note that the cells formed from the myelocytic lineage are produced only in bone marrow, whereas the cells of the lymphocytic lineage (lymphocytes and plasma cells) are produced mainly in the lymph glands, spleen, thymus, tonsils and other lymphoid areas in the bone marrow, gut and elsewhere. Finally, note the differentiation of some of the myelocyte precursors into megakaryocytes, which then fragment into platelets.

Questions for discussion

■ Which factors are involved in the control of white cell production in the bone marrow?

■ What are 'T' and 'B' lymphocytes?

■ What differences can you find between 'T' and 'B' lymphocytes?

Examination 1

When you examined Mrs Evans, you found that she was quite thin and pale. There was a mass in the left side of the abdomen just under the ribs, and marked tenderness to pressure over the 4th thoracic vertebra. The small muscles of the hand were slightly wasted and there was distal weakness in all four limbs. The tendon reflexes were absent and the plantar reflexes were flexor. There was mild diminution of light touch sensation over the hands and feet. There were no detectable abnormalities in the cardiovascular or respiratory systems.

Questions for discussion

■ Why do you think that Mrs Evans is pale and thin?

■ What causes of weight loss could be relevant to Mrs Evans?

■ What do you think the mass in the left side of the abdomen could be?

■ What causes do you know of a vertebra that is tender to pressure?

■ What is the innervation of the small muscles of the hand?

■ What type of neurological disorder do you think that Mrs Evans is suffering from? Make a list of the causes of this type of disorder.

■ Do the examination details give you any more help in formulating a differential diagnosis?

■ Which investigations do you think might be helpful in the case of Mrs Evans?

Activity 10.9

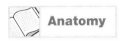 **Anatomy**

▶ Before you examine your partner's abdomen, it is wise to study the size and position of the various abdominal organs.

▶ Ask your partner to strip to the waist and lie supine on an examination table. You are going to examine his abdomen, and in particular his spleen. In the healthy person the spleen is almost never palpable and if the spleen can be felt it usually means that it is enlarged.

▶ Stand on your partner's right side. Observe the abdomen and note whether there are any areas of fullness, scars, distended veins, or evidence of visible peristalsis. Note whether the umbilicus is everted.

▶ Now palpate his abdomen, lightly at first, and then a little more deeply. Use the flat of your hand, and examine each quadrant in turn, feeling for tenderness, guarding, rigidity of the abdomen, and masses. Look at your partner's face while you are doing this, to note whether you are hurting him.

▶ Feel for the liver. Place your right hand on your partner's right iliac fossa, and press firmly but not too deeply. Ask him to take a deep breath in and out, while you feel for any sensation of a structure contacting your right hand.

▶ Repeat the manoeuvre several times, working upwards towards the right costal margin. In a thin person, it may just be possible to feel the liver edge under the ribs.

▶ Now reach right across his abdomen with your left hand and place it over his left costovertebral angle. Lift your left hand upwards slightly to push the spleen towards the anterior abdominal wall. Now place your right hand on your partner's abdomen so that your fingers are extended and pointing horizontally to the left under his left costal margin. Your partner should be asked to take a deep breath in, while you feel for the edge of the spleen to come down onto your fingers.

You should be prepared to press fairly firmly and deeply under a patient's left costal margin in order to palpate a spleen which is enlarged to a minor degree. However, it is important to be gentle in order to avoid rupturing an enlarged spleen. You should start your palpation for the spleen in the right iliac fossa, because the spleen enlarges downwards and medially, and so a very large spleen may reach right across the midline.

▶ Now ask your partner to lie on his right side, and flex his hips and knees slightly. Continue to stand on the right side of the examination couch. Press forward with the fingers of your left hand into your partner's left costovertebral angle (this assists gravity in bringing the spleen closer to the anterior abdominal wall) and press under his left costal margin with the fingertips of your right hand. Again, you should not be able to feel the spleen in this way unless it is enlarged.

Questions for discussion

■ What are the physical signs of an enlarged spleen?

■ What are the physical signs of an enlarged liver?

■ What other physical signs might you find in a person who has an enlarged liver?

■ How would you distinguish between an enlarged spleen and an enlarged left kidney?

■ What causes do you know of an enlarged spleen that might be relevant to Mrs Evans?

■ What else would you examine (apart from the aspects discussed above) if you were performing a complete abdominal examination?

Examination 2

Blood examination of Mrs Evans showed the following:

Haemoglobin	9.5 g dl^{-1}
White cell count	3.0 × 10^9 l^{-1}
Platelet count	90 × 10^9 l^{-1}
Blood film	Red cells normochromic and normocytic. Occasional plasma cells
ESR:	127 mm in the first hour
Plasma urea	12.0 mmol l^{-1}
Plasma calcium	2.7 mmol l^{-1}
Plasma sodium	140 mmol l^{-1}
Plasma potassium	4.0 mmol l^{-1}
Blood glucose	6.4 mmol l^{-1}
Urinalysis	Slight proteinuria only

X-ray of the thoracic spine showed that one pedicle of T4 was missing.

X-ray of the lumbar spine showed that there were several lytic lesions in the vertebral bodies.

Questions for discussion

■ What might be the significance of the missing pedicle at T4 and the lytic lesions in the lumbar vertebral bodies?

■ What do you think of Mrs Evans's haemoglobin, white cell count and platelet count? What type of disease process might cause this blood picture? What symptoms might occur in a patient with this type of blood picture?

■ What causes of a markedly raised ESR do you think are relevant to Mrs Evans?

■ What do you think is the mechanism of Mrs Evans's hypercalcaemia?

■ Now what types of diagnosis would you be considering?

■ Which further investigations might be helpful in clarifying your diagnosis?

■ What relevance do you think that the pulmonary embolus might have to Mrs Evans's condition?

■ Why might Mrs Evans be breathless?

■ What are you going to say to Mrs Evans about her condition?

Activity 10.10

 Pathophysiology

▶ Study the clinical effects of anaemia. Note:

— The effects on blood viscosity and the consequent effects on resistance to blood flow in the peripheral vessels

— The effect of decreased tissue oxygenation on the calibre of peripheral arterioles, and thus on venous return and cardiac output.

One of the major effects of anaemia on the circulation is a substantially increased work load on the heart. In a person with a normal heart, this may not give rise to symptoms. However, if the person has some degree of cardiac insufficiency or ischaemic heart disease, the extra load may be sufficient to produce cardiac failure.

Questions for discussion

- What mechanisms do you know that may produce anaemia?
- How is anaemia classified?
- Can you think of any difficulties with the classification of anaemia?
- What differences are there between Mr Ibbotson's anaemia (Ch. 8) and that of Mrs Evans?

Activity 10.11

- ▶ Collect your urine for a period of 24 hours in a clear glass container.

- ▶ Look at the volume that you have produced, the colour, and whether or not it is frothy (you may find that there is a little froth as soon as you have produced the urine, but this should soon disappear). You will find more activities on urine production in Chapter 13, but for this case consider the fact that Mrs Evans's urine was frothy and there was a small amount of protein in it.

- ▶ Take a small sample (around 10 ml should be sufficient) and place it in a small, clear, heat-proof container such as a test tube.

- ▶ Place the container on a source of heat (a naked flame such as is produced in a Bunsen burner is probably best, but you can improvise) and gradually bring the urine to the boil. Observe the urine for any sign of a precipitate.

- ▶ Let the urine cool and again observe for cloudiness or sediment.

- ▶ Put a little raw egg white into the urine and repeat the boiling procedure. You should find that the urine plus egg white turns cloudy on boiling because of the coagulation of the egg protein with heat. The precipitation should remain when the urine is cooled down to room temperature.

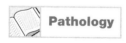 **Pathology**

- ▶ Study the type of protein called a Bence Jones protein.

The characteristic of proteinuria with this protein is that, while a precipitate is formed when the urine is boiled, the precipitate disappears on cooling. Nowadays, this test for Bence Jones proteinuria has been replaced by much more sophisticated laboratory tests such as electrophoresis of the urine, but it is still a useful rapid test if facilities are not available.

The Bence Jones protein is a so-called paraprotein. It is a monoclonal immunoglobulin produced by a proliferation of B lymphocytes when they are relatively mature. On electrophoresis of either urine or serum, an abnormal band is found.

Questions for discussion

■ In which diseases are paraproteins found?

■ What symptoms may paraproteins produce by themselves?

Activity 10.12

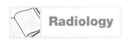 **Radiology**

▶ Study a plain X-ray of the thoracic spine. (There are further details on how to look at a plain radiograph of a vertebra in Ch. 13.) For this case consider particularly the pedicles of the vertebrae. In most of the vertebrae, they appear as white circles on either side of the midline.

Questions for discussion

■ Why do the pedicles appear as white circles on a plain X-ray?

■ Do you notice anything abnormal in this film?

■ What disorders may lead to disappearance of the pedicles?

Examination 3

Mrs Evans underwent some further investigations. Electrophoresis was performed on a sample of her blood, and it was found that there was a paraprotein in the gamma globulin region associated with a decrease in the normal gamma globulin band. A sample of bone marrow was taken from Mrs Evans's sternum and was found to be heavily infiltrated with plasma cells.

Questions for discussion

■ What are plasma cells?

■ What do you think is the diagnosis now?

■ How would you treat Mrs Evans's pain?

Activity 10.13

▶ You will need a small sheet of blotting paper, some different food colourings, a battery and some wire for this activity. Cut the sheet into a strip approximately 2 cm wide and 20 cm long. Fold the strip about 1 cm from one end.

▶ Mix at least two different food colours with water.

▶ Lay the strip horizontally with the folded end dipping into the coloured water (see Fig. 10.1). Observe the coloured liquid moving along the paper.

▶ Wait about 30 minutes. What do you observe?

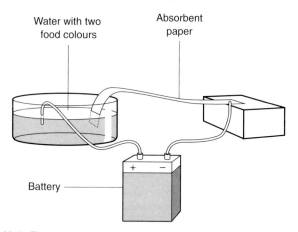

Water with two food colours

Absorbent paper

Battery

Fig. 10.1 Find out what difference a battery makes to the speed of colour separation.

With the colours that I used (red and green), there was a front of faintly green coloured water moving along the paper, while a 'second front' of strong red colour moved along somewhat behind (see Fig. 10.2).

The point about this simple experiment is that it is possible to separate out the two colours which had been mixed.

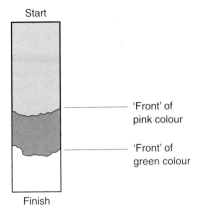

Fig. 10.2 A front of green coloured water, followed by a second front of strong red colour.

Question for discussion

■ Why did the two colours separate?

▶ Now repeat the experiment with the strip of paper soaked in plain water before being dipped in the coloured liquid. You should find that a similar separation of the colours occurs, but the fronts are more diffuse.

▶ Finally, if you have a battery, arrange some wire to the positive and negative poles. Connect the 'start' end of the paper strip to the positive pole and the 'finish' end to the negative pole (see Fig. 10.1).

▶ Repeat the experiment with this arrangement. Is there any difference in the speed at which the colours separate?

Question for discussion

■ On what basis are the colours being separated when there is a battery in the system?

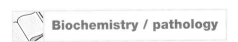

Biochemistry / pathology

▶ Study the technique and uses of electrophoresis. You will note that electrophoresis is usually performed on serum rather than plasma.

Questions for discussion

■ What is the difference between serum and plasma?

■ Why should serum be better than plasma for performing electrophoresis?

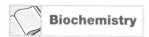 **Biochemistry**

▶ Electrophoresis separates the proteins in blood into distinct bands, depending on their molecular weight and charge. Study the different proteins in normal blood that can be detected by this technique.

▶ Look also at the detection of abnormal proteins, and in particular the paraproteins.

Question for discussion

■ Why must electrophoresis be performed on urine as well as serum if paraprotein secretion is suspected?

Activity 10.14

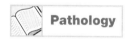 **Pathology**

▶ Study the appearances of a bone marrow biopsy. In particular, look at the appearances of malignant plasma cells in bone marrow. These are large cells which have a 'halo' around the nucleus. A bone marrow appearance such as this is characteristic of multiple myeloma. Note also that in multiple myeloma there is erosion of the surrounding bone.

Questions for discussion

■ How might erosion of the bone be related to Mrs Evans's X-ray appearances?

■ How might bone erosion be related to Mrs Evans's blood calcium result? (See Chs 13 and 14 for further information on calcium metabolism.)

■ What other effects might be produced from infiltration of bone marrow by a malignant process?

Activity 10.15

▶ Study the features of multiple myeloma. This is a malignant process involving the B cells in the bone marrow, the plasma cell being the prevailing cell type.

▶ Look at the effects of the bone marrow infiltration on the surrounding bone, leading to:

— Pain

— Pathological fractures

— X-ray abnormalities

— Hypercalcaemia

— Anaemia

— Suppression of other bone marrow elements.

▶ Look also at the systemic features of the disease, and in particular the effects on the kidney and the nervous system.

Questions for discussion

■ What are the criteria for establishing a diagnosis of multiple myeloma?

■ Which other diseases can give similar clinical and laboratory features to those of multiple myeloma?

■ Which factors adversely affect the prognosis in multiple myeloma?

■ From the information you have been given in this case, what would you estimate Mrs Evans's prognosis to be?

■ What are the objectives of the management of a patient with multiple myeloma?

■ How would you discuss the problem with Mrs Evans?

■ As a manual therapist, what would be your objectives in helping Mrs Evans?

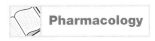 **Pharmacology**

▶ Study the specific drugs used for treating patients with multiple myeloma.

▶ Look in particular at the drug melphalan, which is a nitrogen mustard and one of the class of drugs known as alkylating agents.

The nitrogen mustards were the earliest drugs to be used as cytotoxic chemotherapy. In order to understand fully how cytotoxic agents work, it is necessary to have a knowledge of the cell cycle and the control of cell division.

▶ For this case, look at the mechanism of action of the alkylating agents.

Alkylating agents are so called because they can add alkyl groups to many electronegative groups in the conditions that occur in a living cell. It is thought that they act by preventing the uncoiling of the DNA strand during replication and so preventing cell division.

Questions for discussion

■ For which disorders is melphalan most useful?

■ What side-effects might limit the usefulness of melphalan?

■ Do malignant cells become resistant to the effects of alkylating agents?

Discussion

As mentioned in the introductory remarks to this case, when a person complains of a multitude of seemingly disparate symptoms, it is tempting to attribute them to the product of a psychological problem. It is indeed true that emotional, social or spiritual stress may aggravate and even produce many physical symptoms, and the literature of psychosomatic medicine is ample testimony to this. Nevertheless, it is always important to think of pathological reasons for a person's symptoms so that an appropriate course of action may be pursued and appropriate treatment and prognosis given.

   In the case of Mrs Evans, the shifting nature of the pain, the mild breathlessness, the burning sensations and the abdominal symptoms might all be manifestations of hyperventilation. The loss of weight could also have a psychological basis, as might the thirst and increased frequency of urination (polyuria). However, conditions such as diabetes, renal failure and hypercalcaemia may give rise to thirst and polyuria, and there may be a neurological cause for the burning sensations and weakness. Many cancers are associated with a 'paraneoplastic syndrome' which may include neurological, musculoskeletal and haematological manifestations, and those which either metastasise to bone or which primarily attack bone may give rise to hypercalcaemia. The previous history of a pulmonary embolus should arouse some suspicion. It might have followed an episode of bed rest following pain, or it might be a manifestation of a condition causing a hypercoagulable state of the blood, such as a malignancy (particularly pelvic and pancreatic tumours, leukaemia and multiple myeloma), diabetes and connective tissue disorders.

It is therefore important to perform a thorough physical examination on Mrs Evans. The pallor might suggest that she is anaemic, and this would contribute to her shortness of breath by restricting the amount of oxygen that could be carried in the blood. Anaemia is also a feature of renal failure and cancer, although not usually of diabetes. There are many causes of anaemia and frequently physical examination is not very helpful in resolving the problem. The mass in the left upper quadrant of the abdomen might be an enlarged spleen. The list of causes of an enlarged spleen is at least as large as that of anaemia, but in the UK infections, connective tissue disorders, haemolytic anaemias, malignancy (including lymphoma and leukaemia), cardiac failure and portal hypertension are the most likely reasons. In Mrs Evans, the physical examination showed no evidence of heart failure or portal hypertension, and there was no fever, making infection less likely. The neurological signs suggest a sensorimotor peripheral neuropathy, for which there is again an extensive list of causes, including drugs, alcohol, connective tissue disorders, diabetes, thyroid disorders, infections and malignancy.

Despite the apparently endless list of different conditions that might be operating in Mrs Evans, a few relatively simple investigations will help to narrow the field down quite considerably. A full blood count will confirm anaemia and demonstrate the type, and will also demonstrate any abnormalities in the numbers of white cells and platelets. A blood film may demonstrate abnormal cells, such as immature white cells in leukaemia or some plasma cells in multiple myeloma. A raised ESR will give a non-specific hint that an inflammatory process is occurring. A fasting blood glucose level will confirm or exclude diabetes mellitus. Urea and electrolyte levels ('U+E') help to determine whether there is any renal damage or disorder of calcium metabolism, and examination of the urine will show if there is any blood, protein, sugar or bilirubin. An X-ray of the thoracic spine may show osteoporosis or bone destruction.

The results show that Mrs Evans is indeed anaemic, and the blood film shows some plasma cells but no immature white cells. Leukaemia is thus unlikely but multiple myeloma is a strong possibility. The normal blood sugar makes diabetes unlikely. The U+E shows a mildly raised urea, indicating some renal dysfunction, and a raised calcium level. This could indicate a cancer metastasising to the bones or a disease which primarily attacks bone, such as multiple myeloma. Connective tissue disorders commonly cause renal damage but do not generally give rise to hypercalcaemia. The X-ray shows total destruction of bone; this is generally due to either infection or neoplasm. Infection could be with tuberculosis or pyogenic organisms. However, there is no fever and tuberculosis tends to destroy the vertebral bodies rather than the pedicles. Also, the fact that Mrs Evans felt the pain in a number of areas would make bone tuberculosis less likely. A malignant infiltration of the bone could be due to secondary invasion from an undetectable breast or lung primary tumour, or again it could be due to a disease such as leukaemia or multiple myeloma. The anaemia and very high ESR would fit with any of these possibilities, but the presence of plasma cells in the peripheral blood is very suggestive of multiple myeloma. Bone pain in this disorder is often very severe, especially if there are pathological fractures.

Further investigation should include electrophoresis of serum and urine to determine whether there is a monoclonal band. A chest X-ray and a Mantoux test will show whether there is any active tuberculosis and a skeletal survey is needed to look for other sites of bone lesions. A bone marrow specimen should be obtained and examined for evidence of infiltration by myeloma, leukaemia or secondary cancer.

As far as the manual therapist is concerned, physical treatment is unlikely to affect the severity of the pain of multiple myeloma. Local soft tissue work may slightly improve the patient's sense of comfort, but since the pain has its origin in the bone itself, is unlikely to be of more than temporary benefit. It is important to maintain mobility in the spine, but exercises should be used sparingly because of the risk of pathological fracture. Any high-velocity techniques are absolutely contraindicated for the same reason.

The major application of manual therapy is in treating secondary dysfunctions which are causing pain but are not part of the primary pathological process. This may give valuable relief to the patient and may result in a reduced requirement for powerful analgesics. Trigger point therapy and acupuncture would be appropriate for Mrs Evans.

FURTHER READING

Dimopoulos M A, Palumbo A, Delasalle K B, Alexanian R 1994 Primary plasma cell leukaemia. British Journal of Haematology 88: 754–759

Moscinski L C, Ballester O F 1994 Recent progress in multiple myeloma. Haematological Oncology 12: 111–123

Study objectives

After studying this case with its associated activities and questions, you should have a reasonable knowledge of the following areas:

1. Surface anatomy of structures around the ankle and foot
2. Anatomy of the lower end of the tibia and fibula
3. Anatomy of the talus
4. Attachments and functions of the ligaments of the ankle
5. Functional anatomy of the ankle joint and the tibiofibular joints
6. Attachments, actions, blood and nerve supply of muscles acting on the ankle joint
7. Arterial supply to lower leg and ankle
8. Venous drainage of lower leg and ankle
9. Nerve supply to lower leg and ankle
10. Testing active, passive and resisted movements of the ankle
11. Biomechanics of the gait cycle in walking and running
12. Examination of the fingers and toes for clubbing
13. Causes of clubbing of the fingers and toes
14. Clinical features of a joint effusion
15. Causes of a joint effusion
16. Differential diagnosis of ankle pain
17. X-ray features of long bones
18. X-ray features of hypertrophic pulmonary osteoarthropathy (HPOA)
19. Biology of malignant transformation of cells.

Background

Theresa McDonald, a 60-year-old housewife, used to be proud of her feet. In her youth, she had been a dancer and at school she had won a local 'lovely legs' competition. She had always been active and went for walks of at least 5 miles on most weekends. However, over the 4 or 5 months prior to her first consultation with you, she had experienced increasing pain in both ankles and to a lesser extent, both knees. It was the ankle pain that was particularly annoying, but she felt that her general practitioner was not really getting to the root of the matter. He had examined her ankles twice and had pronounced her to be free of arthritis. Nevertheless, he had started her on a non-steroidal anti-inflammatory drug, which had produced a little improvement in her condition. She had pressed the general practitioner for referral to the local orthopaedic clinic, but the waiting time for this was at least 9 months for non-urgent cases and she did not feel that she could wait that long.

The history that you initially elicited from Mrs McDonald was that of pain and tenderness in both ankles and knees, with no radiation up the legs or into the feet. The pain was worse in the mornings and was associated with marked stiffness which lasted at least half an hour before it eased with movement.

Questions for discussion

- What diagnostic possibilities occur to you at this stage?
- What further questions would you like to ask Mrs McDonald?

On further questioning, Mrs McDonald told you that the pain felt like a 'deep bone pain' and was worse on standing. However, it never really seemed to completely ease off, and in fact often woke her up in the night. It was beginning to affect her walking, so that she had felt unable to complete her weekly trip for the past month or so. She had no complaint of swelling of the ankles, but she felt as though the skin was very tight. General enquiry revealed that Mrs McDonald had previously been in very good health, but had lost approximately 5 kg over the previous 3 months with no appreciable loss of appetite. She had a smoker's cough, having been a lifelong smoker of at least 20 cigarettes a day, but this had not noticeably changed and she was not breathless. In fact, she felt that 'if only you could fix her feet, everything would be OK'.

Questions for discussion

■ Does the pain sound musculoskeletal in origin?

■ Are there any worrying features in the history?

■ On which areas would you concentrate in the physical examination?

Activity 11.1

▶ Ask your partner to remove his shoes, socks and trousers for this activity. On your partner's foot and ankle, identify the following structures:

— Medial malleolus

— Lateral malleolus

— Talus

— Calcaneus

— Peroneal tubercle of calcaneus

— Medial tubercle of calcaneus

— Cuboid

— Medial cuneiform

— 1st metatarsal

— 5th metatarsal

— Posterior tibial artery

— Dorsalis pedis artery

— Tendo calcaneus

— Tendon of peroneus longus

— Tendon of peroneus brevis

— Tendon of tibialis posterior

— Tendon of flexor digitorum longus

— Flexor retinaculum

— Superior extensor retinaculum

— Inferior extensor retinaculum.

Activity 11.2

▶ Your partner should still have bare legs for this activity. Ask him to lie supine on an examination couch. Note:

— The position of the foot relative to the lower leg

— Whether the feet face directly forwards in the parasagittal plane or whether your partner is 'pigeon-toed'

— Whether there is any angulation of the big toe (hallux) on the foot to form a hallux valgus, more commonly known as a 'bunion'.

▶ Grasp your partner's right leg just above the ankle with your left hand, and his right foot just below the ankle with your right hand.

▶ Perform the following passive movements on your partner's foot:

— Plantarflexion

— Dorsiflexion

— Inversion

— Eversion

— Adduction

— Abduction

— Pronation (a combination of plantarflexion, inversion and adduction)

— Supination (a combination of dorsiflexion, eversion and abduction).

▶ Repeat these movements with your partner's right knee flexed to 90°.

▶ Ask your partner to perform all the movements described above without your help.

Questions for discussion

■ What differences did you find in the range of passive movements when the knee was flexed compared with when the leg was straight?

■ How do you account for any differences that you found?

- Why is it important to assess the passive range of motion of the foot by measuring the movement of the calcaneus rather than that of the forefoot?
- Are there any differences between the passive and active ranges of movement? How do you account for any differences that you found?

▶ Now test the active movements of the feet. Ask your partner to perform the movements described above while you try to resist the movement. (It will be a good exercise for you to discover for yourself the best grips to allow you to resist each of the movements.)

Activity 11.3

▶ You will need a plumb line for this activity. Ask your partner to sit so that his legs are hanging free over the edge of the examination couch. Drop the plumb line from the middle of his patella and note where the lower end falls in relationship to the foot. It should touch the foot between the 1st and 2nd toes.

Question for discussion

- What might be the causes of the plumb line falling medial to the foot when the upper end is in the middle of the patella?

▶ Ask your partner to stand. Observe the feet and ankles in this position.

▶ Check the concavity of the longitudinal arch of the foot.

▶ If your partner does not have a 'flat foot', examine someone you know does have one when you get a chance.

▶ Look at a footprint made by your partner and one by someone with a flat foot.

Question for discussion

- How might 'knock-knees' (genu valgum) contribute to the production of a flat foot?

Activity 11.4

▶ Ask your partner to walk around the room. (There are more activities in Ch. 3 regarding the muscles around the hip joint that are involved in walking.)

► Observe the movement of one leg during the different phases of walking.

► Observe the two main phases of walking (termed the 'gait cycle'):
  — Stance, i.e. the leg is weight-bearing
  — Swing, i.e. the leg is off the ground.

► Observe the fact that there is a small part of the cycle in which both feet are weight-bearing.

► Note particularly the position of the foot on the floor during the stance phase. The heel strikes the floor, the foot then flattens, then the ankle rises and the toes push the foot off the floor.

► Note the following features of a normal gait cycle (take your time):
  — Rotation of the pelvis forwards with the swinging leg and backwards with the stance leg
  — Tilting of the pelvis downwards on the swinging side and upwards on the stance side
  — Rotation of the femur and tibia internally during the swing and first half of the stance phase, and externally during the second half of the stance phase
  — Flexion and extension of the knee as the leg passes through the stance phase
  — Plantarflexion and dorsiflexion of the ankle as the leg passes through the stance phase
  — Stretching of the plantar fascia during the stance phase
  — Dorsiflexion of the toes during the push off of the weight-bearing leg.

Questions for discussion

■ What proportion of the gait cycle is swing, and what proportion is stance?

■ For what proportion of the gait cycle are both feet on the ground (double-leg phase)?

■ What happens to the body's centre of gravity during the gait cycle?

■ How do pelvic rotation and pelvic tilt affect the movement of the body's centre of gravity during walking?

■ How do the different elements of the gait cycle interact to conserve energy during walking?

■ What do you think would happen to the gait cycle if there was an arthritic restriction of
  - one hip
  - both hips
  - one knee
  - both knees
  - one ankle
  - both ankles?

▶ Now ask your partner to jog around the room. Observe the gait cycle as in walking.

▶ Repeat the observations with your partner running around the room. Note particularly the relative proportions of the swing and stance phases, and the proportion of the cycle in which both feet are off the floor.

▶ Observe the following in jogging and running:
  — The range of motion of the hips, knees and ankles as the stride length increases
  — The degree of knee flexion
  — The angle of the ankle on the foot during the stance phase
  — The impact of the foot on the floor.

Questions for discussion

■ Why do you think that the following injuries are common in runners and joggers
  - painful heel pads
  - strained hamstring muscles
  - plantar fasciitis
  - stress fractures
  - 'shin splints'
  - chondromalacia patellae?

Activity 11.5

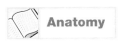 **Anatomy**

▶ Study the functional anatomy of the ankle joint. (Do not study the detailed anatomy of the foot for this case, although it is clearly difficult to separate the functions of the ankle joint from those of the other foot joints.) First, study the bones that make up the posterior part of the foot and the lower end of the tibia and fibula. Note:

— The general shape of the talus with its body, neck and head

— The superior surface of the talus, and how its convex saddle shape allows it to glide under the tibia during ankle motion.

▶ Look at the reciprocal concavity on the inferior surface of the tibia.

▶ Note also how the talus is gripped by the medial and lateral malleoli of the tibia and fibula respectively, and study the almost plane medial surface and concave lateral surface of the body of the talus.

▶ Note particularly the fact that the groove on top of the talus does not lie in a sagittal plane. This is because the medial malleolus is anterior to the lateral malleolus. The neck of the talus thus faces anteriorly and medially.

▶ Study the axis of rotation of the talus between the malleoli, and note that it passes through the lower end of the fibula but below the end of the tibia, and is inclined at about 15° to the sagittal plane, producing a small degree of external rotation.

▶ Study the ligaments around the ankle. Note:

— The two collateral ligaments attached to the corresponding malleolus and to the posterior tarsal bones, and the anterior and posterior ligaments of the ankle, which are just thickenings of the joint capsule

— That the lateral collateral ligament comprises
  - anterior talofibular ligament
  - calcaneofibular ligament
  - posterior talofibular ligament

— That the medial collateral ligament comprises
  - anterior talotibial ligament
  - posterior talotibial ligament
  - deltoid ligament.

▶ Study the attachments of these ligaments, and note how their arrangement influences the anteroposterior and lateral stability of the ankle joint.

Questions for discussion

■ The total range of dorsiflexion and plantarflexion at the ankle joint is approximately 140°. How does the anatomy of the bones of the ankle joint determine this value?

■ Which bony, ligamentous and muscular factors limit plantarflexion and dorsiflexion at the ankle joint?

■ How do the following contribute to the anteroposterior stability of the ankle joint:
  – gravity
  – the anterior and posterior margins of the tibial surface
  – the collateral ligaments?

■ Which ligament is affected in an inversion sprain of the ankle?

Activity 11.6

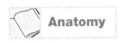 **Anatomy**

▶ The tibiofibular joints and their associated ligaments should be studied next. It is logical to study the superior tibiofibular joint as well as the inferior joint at this stage, because it is mechanically linked to the ankle rather than the knee. Note the superior tibiofibular joint, with its oval articular facets. It is a plane joint, with the tibial facet facing posteriorly, inferiorly and laterally, and articulating with the fibular facet. Note the close relationship of the popliteus muscle, the lateral collateral ligament of the knee and the tendon of the biceps femoris muscle to the joint.

▶ Study the anterior and posterior ligaments of the superior tibiofibular joint.

▶ Look at the inferior tibiofibular joint. This contains no articular cartilage, and the two bones are separated by fibro-fatty tissue. Note:
  — The rough, concave tibial facet and the fibular facet which may be slightly concave, plane or slightly convex
  — The close relationship of the fibular articular facet and the lateral collateral ligament of the ankle to the joint
  — The anterior ligament of the joint running inferiorly and laterally, the thicker posterior ligament and the deep transverse tibiofibular ligament, and how the ligaments contribute to the socket of the ankle joint
  — The interosseous ligament.

▶ Study the attachments of the interosseous ligament and the direction of its fibres.

Questions for discussion

■ The body of the talus widens from posterior to anterior. How does this fact affect the inferior tibiofibular joint during plantarflexion and dorsiflexion of the ankle joint?

■ How does separation and approximation of the medial and lateral malleoli during plantarflexion and dorsiflexion cause axial rotation of the lateral malleolus?

■ How does rotation of the lateral malleolus cause vertical movement of the fibula during ankle movements?

■ How does ankle movement cause movement of the superior tibiofibular joint?

Activity 11.7

▶ Ask your partner to repeat the active and resisted movements of the ankle in Activity 11.2.

▶ Once you have done this, ask your partner to stand with his weight evenly distributed between both feet, and then close his eyes.

▶ Observe how much he sways forwards and backwards and from side to side.

▶ Ask him to deliberately sway backwards slightly, and note which muscles become active.

▶ Repeat this with your partner swaying forwards and to one side.

▶ Ask your partner to open his eyes and stand on one leg for a short while, and then ask him to close his eyes. In each case, observe the amount of sway of the body.

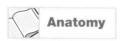 **Anatomy**

▶ Study the muscles that produce the movements and help to maintain stability in the upright posture. Concentrate on the extrinsic muscles of the foot and ankle, i.e. those that originate away from the foot and ankle but act upon their joints.

▶ Study the attachments, trigger points, nerve supply and actions of the following muscles:

— Gastrocnemius
— Soleus
— Tibialis anterior
— Tibialis posterior
— Flexor digitorum longus
— Extensor digitorum longus
— Flexor hallucis longus
— Extensor hallucis longus
— Peroneus longus
— Peroneus brevis.

▶ Note that during relaxed standing, only the gastrocnemius and soleus muscles are tonically active, with ligaments providing the rest of the support.

Question for discussion

■ Which muscles are active during standing on one leg?

▶ Study the nerve supply to the structures of the lower leg and ankle. You should already have looked at the nerve supply to the extrinsic muscles of the area, but now study the arrangement of the nerves in the leg and which nerves come off at which level. This will determine the loss of motor and sensory function that may occur when an injury is sustained at a particular level.

▶ Study the continuation of the sciatic nerve into the tibial and the common peroneal nerves, and the emergence of the branches of these nerves to the various muscles.

Activity 11.8

▶ With your partner lying supine on an examination couch, look at the arterial supply on his lower leg. Feel the pulsations of the posterior tibial artery behind the medial malleolus deep to the flexor retinaculum, and the dorsalis pedis artery on the dorsum of the foot about halfway between the medial and lateral malleoli.

▶ Now ask your partner to stand upright and observe the veins in his leg.

▶ Look at the venous arch on the dorsum of the foot, and follow it laterally and medially to the short and long saphenous veins. (There are further details regarding the venous circulation in Ch. 2.)

 Anatomy

▶ Study the arterial supply and venous drainage of the lower part of the leg.

▶ Follow the course of the anterior tibial artery between the tibia and fibula, passing down on the anterior surface of the interosseous membrane.

The anterior tibial artery supplies branches to the muscles of the anterior compartment of the leg and gives rise to the medial and lateral malleolar arteries which supply the ankle. The dorsalis pedis artery is just a continuation of the anterior tibial artery as it passes in front of the ankle joint.

▶ Now follow the posterior tibial artery descending in the calf to supply the muscles of the posterior compartment before passing into the foot deep to the flexor retinaculum and dividing into the medial and lateral plantar arteries.

▶ Study the venous drainage of the lower leg (see also Ch. 2). Note the superficial and deep systems of veins, and the communication between the two systems via the perforating veins.

Question for discussion

■ What is the 'muscle pump' in the lower limb and what is its significance?

Having considered the anatomy of the structures that could possibly give rise to pain in the lower leg and ankle, it is time to consider Mrs McDonald's problem again, and in particular the findings on physical examination.

Examination 1

On physical examination, Mrs McDonald did not look particularly well, and was clearly in some pain. There was no sign of pallor, jaundice or cyanosis, but there was marked nicotine staining of several fingers of the right hand. There was also gross clubbing affecting the fingers and toes. Examination of the hands otherwise showed no

abnormality, and in particular there were no signs of
arthritis. There was tenderness in both legs just above the
ankle anteriorly, and there were signs of a small effusion in
both ankle joints. There was a distinct impression that the
ankles and lower legs were warm, although there was no
discolouration or oedema of the legs. Ankle movements
were not restricted when you examined them, although Mrs
McDonald commented that if you had examined them first
thing in the morning, then there would have been a lot of
stiffness. Abdominal examination was normal and there
was no neurological deficit. There were no abnormal
physical signs in the cardiovascular or respiratory systems.
Examination of the spine revealed no significant restriction,
and examination of the rest of the musculoskeletal system
did not show any further joint restrictions or effusions.

Questions for discussion

- What are the causes of clubbing of the fingers and/or toes?
  Make a list.
- Which of the causes of clubbing do you think might be
  applicable to Mrs McDonald's problem?
- What are the signs of an effusion into the ankle joint?
- What causes can you think of for an effusion into the ankle
  joint? Which of these may be relevant to Mrs McDonald?
- What special investigations do you think might be appropriate
  for further clarification of the problem?

Activity 11.9

▶ You could perform this activity on your partner's toes as well
as his fingers, but it is just a little easier to use the fingers and
all comments apply equally to the toes. Look at your partner's
fingers, and observe the nail beds closely.
▶ Ask your partner to flex his index finger at the proximal and
distal interphalangeal joints. Get a straight edge (a ruler will
do) and place it along the dorsal surface of the distal part of
the finger including the nail. Now look at the finger from the
side. You should find that there is a space between the nail
bed and the straight edge.

▶ Ask your partner to place the dorsal surfaces of both index fingers together. It will again help to have the fingers flexed and just the distal parts of the fingers touching. Again observe the finger from the side, and note that there is a diamond-shaped space between the nail beds.

▶ Now place two straight edges so that they meet at the base of the nail and are aligned along the nail and the distal part of the finger (Fig. 11.1).

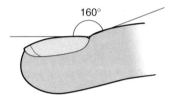

Fig. 11.1 A normal (not clubbed) finger.

▶ Measure the angle between the two straight edges. In a normal person, the angle should be approximately 160°.

▶ Now place the tips of both your index fingers on either side of the nail of your partner's index finger. Try to rock his nail from side to side, and note how 'spongy' the feeling is.

When the nails are clubbed, there is an increased sponginess in the feeling when you press on the nails, and it is easier to rock them from side to side. The angle between the nail bed and the finger increases to 180° or more (see Fig. 11.2).

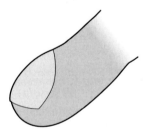

Fig. 11.2 A clubbed finger.

With clubbing, the diamond-shaped space between the fingers disappears, and with advanced clubbing the ends of the fingers become bulbous and resemble drumsticks.

There is often much discussion over whether or not a particular patient has clubbing. If there is doubt, it may be better to assume that it is present and investigate accordingly, particularly if there are other features suggestive of relevant pathology.

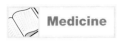 **Medicine**

▶ Look at the causes of clubbing.

You will find that there are many pathological causes, particularly related to the cardiovascular and respiratory systems, but it can also be associated with inflammatory bowel disease and cirrhosis of the liver. It is important to remember that clubbing may also be congenital and not associated with any pathology.

Your textbooks of pathology or physiology may not give an explanation of the mechanism of production of clubbing of the fingers. All that seems to be known is that there is an increased blood flow through the fingers and that cutting the vagus nerve may prevent clubbing.

Examination 2

Mrs McDonald had a blood sample taken. The results of the analysis were as follows:

Haemoglobin	11.0 g dl^{-1}
White cell count	7.5 × 10^9 l^{-1}
ESR	36 mm in first hour
Urea and electrolytes	Normal
Liver function tests	Normal
Rheumatoid factor	Positive at a titre of 1/64

Chest X-ray showed a rounded opacity in the left mid-zone. X-ray of the ankle showed a 1 mm wide line shadow running parallel to the bone, indicating periostitis and new bone formation.

Questions for discussion

■ Now what do you think is the probable diagnosis?

■ Are there any other investigations that might help to confirm or clarify your thoughts about the diagnosis?

Activity 11.10

▶ Take a polo mint or similar annular object. Look at it end-on.

▶ Place the mint on a sheet of graph paper and draw round both the outer and inner margins of the mint.

▶ Measure the thickness of the solid part of the mint at various positions.

You will have noted that the thickest part of the annulus occurs at the margin of the inner ring. It will be useful to make some quantification of this.

▶ Consider the annulus shown in Figure 11.3.

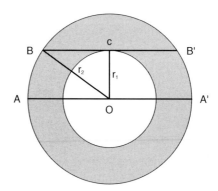

Fig. 11.3 Annulus.

The radius of the inner ring is r_1 and the radius of the outer ring is r_2. Look at the line A–O–A′ at the centre of the annulus. The thickness of the shaded portion is clearly $2(r_2 - r_1)$. Now look at the line B–C–B′ at the margin of the inner ring. The triangle OCB is a right-angled triangle with hypotenuse OB equal to r_2 and length of one side OC equal to r_1.

Using Pythagoras's theorem:

$$BC^2 = OB^2 - OC^2$$
$$= r_2{}^2 - r_1{}^2$$

Thus the thickness of B–B′ is equal to $2\sqrt{(r_2{}^2 - r_1{}^2)}$

It is then a matter of straightforward algebra to calculate that the ratio of B–B′ to the shaded portion of A–A′ is equal to:

$$\sqrt{\frac{(r_2 + r_1)}{(r_2 - r_1)}}$$

Consider the implications of this calculation. It may be best to try a few actual numbers first, especially if you are not very good at 'seeing' things in mathematical formulae. First of all, try $r_2 = 2$, 5 and 8 with r_1 fixed at 10 (you need not worry about units for this calculation, since you are looking at a ratio, and the units will cancel out). You should find that the ratios work out at 1.2, 1.7 and 3. In other words, the larger the hole relative to the diameter of the annulus, the greater is the relative thickness at the margin of the inner ring.

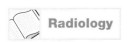
Radiology

▶ Now study a normal radiograph of the tibia and fibula.

When studying plain X-rays, it is important to think three-dimensionally. Long bones such as the tibia and fibula are relatively easy to analyse but still give interesting clues to the study of X-rays of bones in general.

There are two main factors that influence the density of the shadow of a radio-opaque material on the X-ray plate:

— The density of the material
— The distance that the beam has to travel through it.

In a long bone the cortical bone is much denser than the cancellous bone of the medulla. The situation then becomes analogous to that analysed above for the annulus.

Questions for discussion

■ Using the analysis given above for the annulus, can you estimate the thickness of the cortex of the bone relative to the total diameter of the bone for

  – the tibia
  – the fibula?

■ How would you expect the density of the shadow to vary from the centre to the periphery of the tibia?

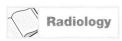
Radiology

▶ Look at a radiograph of a tibia and fibula showing the condition known as hypertrophic pulmonary osteoarthropathy.

Question for discussion

■ What do you notice about the periphery of the tibia in this condition?

 Medicine / radiology

▶ Study the condition known as hypertrophic pulmonary osteoarthropathy (HPOA). Note that this condition involves periostitis, clubbing of fingers and toes which may be very marked, and arthropathy.

HPOA is usually associated with carcinoma of the bronchus, but there are other pulmonary abnormalities which may give rise to the condition, such as benign or malignant pleural tumours, empyema, fibrosing alveolitis, chronic lung sepsis and bronchiectasis. Although the condition is termed 'pulmonary', there are a number of causes which originate remote from the lung, such as cyanotic heart disease, ulcerative colitis, and thyroid disease.

Questions for discussion

■ Which bones are commonly affected by HPOA?
■ Which cause of HPOA do you think applies to Mrs McDonald?

In the X-ray, the long bones have an 'elm-bark' appearance due to the periosteal reaction. Clinically, the affected areas may be hot and tender and sometimes there is associated oedema.

Examination 3

A sample of Mrs McDonald's sputum was analysed under the microscope and found to contain adenocarcinoma cells. Fibre optic bronchoscopy showed no abnormality. A bone scan showed increased uptake of the isotope in the distal parts of both tibiae and fibulae.

Questions for discussion

■ The diagnosis should be clear to you now, but why might the bronchoscopy have yielded a negative result?
■ What histological types of lung cancer can you think of?

- What is the prognosis of adenocarcinoma relative to the other histological type of lung cancer?
- Given the information that you have about Mrs McDonald, revise how you would distinguish between rheumatoid arthritis, HPOA and secondary malignant deposits in the tibiae and fibulae.
- What do you think ought to be done for Mrs McDonald?
- Is there any way that a manual therapist could be of help in this case?
- What advice on smoking would you give Mrs McDonald?

Activity 11.11

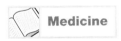 **Medicine**

▶ Study some aspects of the biology of cancer. There are further details about the spread of tumours in Chapter 6, but for this case you should concentrate on how a normal cell can be transformed into a cancerous one. It has to be stated at the outset that this is an incompletely understood subject, but quite a lot is known about the factors that are associated with cancer.

Questions for discussion

- Make a list of factors that you know are associated with an increased risk of developing cancer.
- Are any of the factors that you have listed relevant to Mrs McDonald?

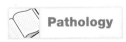 **Pathology**

▶ Study what is termed the 'multistep theory' of neoplasia. The implications of such a theory are not only that multiple stages are involved before a normal cell becomes a cancerous cell, but also that many of the factors that we say 'cause' cancer are only one influence on the total process. Look at the stages of initiation and promotion of carcinogenesis.

Questions for discussion

■ What are the differences between
  - a complete and an incomplete carcinogen
  - a direct and an indirect carcinogen?

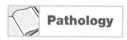 **Pathology**

▶ Now study the link between genes and cancer.

This link is important even in non-inherited cancers, since it is believed that the factors that you have noted above as being associated with cancer act through common genetic pathways to produce a cell which has been transformed from a normal into a malignant one. When you looked in your textbook, you should have found that there are molecules known as oncogenes which can transform normal cells into malignant ones. The normal gene from which the oncogene is derived is called a proto-oncogene (p-onc), and that there are endogenous (c-onc) and exogenous (v-onc) oncogenes.

Questions for discussion

■ What is a gene?
■ What functions of genes do you know?
■ What is a chromosome?
■ What is DNA?
■ How do changes in the structure of DNA cause disease?

Some of the exogenous oncogenes are similar to normal cellular genes while others are totally different. Proto-oncogenes in a normal cell may be become transformed into oncogenes either by spontaneous mutation, or under the influence of factors such as radiation, chemicals or viruses. This changes the structure of the DNA so that the controls on cell growth are altered.

Questions for discussion

■ How may oncogenes act through
  - altering production of cell growth factors
  - altering the structure of growth factor receptors on the cell surface
  - altering 'messenger' molecules which travel between the receptors and the cell nucleus

– altering the nuclear proteins associated with control of the cell cycle?

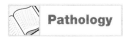
Pathology

▶ As an added complication, look at the proteins called suppressor proteins that normally inhibit cell growth.

In some cancers, the genes that code for these proteins are deficient. For example, the suppressor protein p53 is carried on the short arm of chromosome 17. In some cases of breast cancer, part of the short arm of chromosome 17 is lost, the suppressor protein is not made, and so growth of some cells is not regulated normally.

The study of the cellular mechanisms involved in production of cancers is still at an early stage, but it is hoped that elucidation of genetic mechanisms such as briefly outlined above will yield exciting new insights.

Discussion

Mrs McDonald's main complaint was of pain in the ankles and knees. There was also morning stiffness, and she had responded to a certain extent to a non-steroidal anti-inflammatory drug. Physical examination showed small effusions in both ankles, and the blood tests showed the presence of rheumatoid factor in low titre. The obvious diagnosis on this information would seem to be rheumatoid arthritis. However, there are several factors that should be considered before concluding that this is the diagnosis. First, there is the loss of weight. Although this may occur with any acute arthritis, the possibility of a malignant process must always be borne in mind, especially since a polyarthritis may precede any more specific symptoms and signs of a tumour. Mrs McDonald was a smoker of many years' standing, and despite the absence of specific respiratory symptoms, a lung cancer must remain a possibility.

This suspicion is reinforced by the presence of clubbing of the fingers and toes. You should have made a list of the causes of clubbing, and you will have noted that the commonest cause is carcinoma of the bronchus. It may occur with any histological type of lung cancer, but is most often associated with squamous cell tumours.

The X-ray taken of Mrs McDonald's lower legs and ankles show periostitis and new bone formation. This is characteristic of hypertrophic pulmonary osteoarthropathy. This is related to clubbing and also occurs most commonly with carcinoma of the bronchus, but may also occur with other causes of clubbing. Clinically, the patient complains of painful joints, particularly wrists, elbows, knees and ankles, which may be accompanied by morning stiffness and may show a response to non-steroidal anti-inflammatory drugs. You can see that it is very easy to confuse this condition with rheumatoid arthritis, particularly since about 10% of people over the age of 60 years have a low titre of rheumatoid factor. In Mrs McDonald's case, this finding only serves to add to the diagnostic confusion.

Another potential source of confusion is with bony metastases from a primary cancer such as lung, breast or kidney. A high quality bone scan will be able to distinguish metastases from HPOA, since in the former the isotope is concentrated in the centre of the bones whereas HPOA shows deposition around the cortex.

Many lung cancers, and particularly adenocarcinomas, arise in the periphery of the lung, and thus may reach a large size before causing symptoms. They are often encountered on routine chest X-ray for a problem unrelated to respiratory symptoms. In Mrs McDonald's case, there is a further diagnostic confusion between a tumour mass and a lesion due to a pulmonary manifestation of rheumatoid arthritis. The sputum cytology in Mrs McDonald showed malignant cells, but often this is not the case, and diagnosis may have to be made by tissue biopsy, either via the bronchi or through the skin.

A fairly high proportion of patients with adenocarcinoma prove to be suitable for surgery to remove the tumour mass, and it is often possible to eradicate the tumour. A further feature is that the HPOA and clubbing often regress after removal of the tumour.

Once the diagnosis has been made, it is not worth spending time on trying to alleviate the pain of HPOA using manual therapy. Soft tissue work will just exacerbate the inflammatory process, and working on the muscles and joints by stretching or manipulation will have little beneficial effect. Once the tumour mass has been removed, the inflammation may begin to subside and soft tissue work may then give some relief.

FURTHER READING

Sansores R H, Villalba-Caloca J, Ramirez-Venegas A et al 1995 Reversal of digital clubbing after lung transplantation. Chest 107: 283–285

Mr John Newman

After studying this case with its associated activities and questions, you should have a reasonable knowledge of the following areas:

1. Surface anatomy of structures in the anterior thorax
2. Surface markings of heart and lungs
3. Surface markings of heart valves
4. Surface markings of major blood vessels attached to the heart
5. Relations of the heart in the chest
6. Histology of cardiac muscle
7. Histology of the conducting system of the heart
8. Anatomy of the coronary blood vessels
9. Control of coronary blood flow
10. Nerve supply to the heart
11. Electrical events of the cardiac cycle
12. Concept of vectors
13. Basic ideas about the formation of the electrocardiograph (ECG)
14. Mechanical events of the cardiac cycle
15. Control of the pumping action of the heart
16. Starling's law of the heart
17. Examination of the heart
18. Types of heart murmur
19. Causes of the various heart murmurs
20. Relationship between stress and heart disease
21. Causes of anterior chest pain
22. Causes of angina.

Background

John Henry Newman was not a happy man. At the age of 49, he had been vicar of a small parish in the country for the past 9 years and although you could not say that life was boring, he never felt that he had fulfilled his potential. In fact, he had started taking on more and more responsibilities over the year or so before he came to see you, and was working from early morning to late in the evening on paperwork for these. His family were complaining that they never saw him, and that he had changed from being a happy-go-lucky family man into an intense being who was always having to rush off to some meeting or other. He felt that, having come relatively late into the priesthood, he had to make up for lost time, so to speak.

The reason he turned up on your doorstep was that for the past 3 months he had noticed some tightness across the front of his chest, and also to a lesser extent between the shoulder blades. The chest pain seemed to extend across the top of the left shoulder and down the inner aspect of the left arm, and he felt some pins and needles in some of the fingers of the left hand. Curiously enough, these sensations were most apparent when he was working under pressure, and particularly when he felt that he was not in control of the situation. Since you were not one of his parishioners and he did not want to discuss certain matters with his general practitioner, he decided that you were the best person from whom to seek advice and possibly treatment.

Questions for discussion

- Do you have an idea of what might be the most likely cause of Mr Newman's symptoms?
- What other causes can you think of for these symptoms?
- What other questions would you ask Mr Newman?

On further questioning, Mr Newman told you that the pain was made worse after a meal or when he went out in the cold weather, but did not seem to be related to posture. It was not aggravated by deep inspiration. He was not breathless, nor did his feet swell, and he had no cough or wheeze. He told you that he smoked about 20 cigarettes a day, and that this had been steadily increasing over the past year or so with the self-imposed pressure of his work.

In the past, Mr Newman had suffered a bout of what was diagnosed as rheumatic fever, but had made a good recovery from this. He had had no other illnesses.

Questions for discussion

- Does the history give you any further clue as to the diagnosis in Mr Newman's case?
- What features of the physical examination would you concentrate on?

Activity 12.1

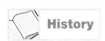 History

▶ Find out about John Henry Newman. Note that he was a prominent figure in the Oxford Movement in the early 19th century. At that time there was a great deal of turmoil, with the industrial revolution and scientific discoveries, and questions were being asked about the nature of the Church of England . . .

I could go on, but this is not a book on the church. However, there is a point to be made here. If you were a physicist and your name were Einstein, just think of the expectations that people would have of your scientific ability. You would feel under great pressure to fulfil those expectations, and an inability to do so might put you under a lot of stress. The John Henry Newman of the 19th century was a very famous figure in the church, and our Mr Newman may well have felt that he was being driven to emulate his illustrious namesake. As a manual therapist, you may need to know a bit about all subjects to understand what makes people act the way they do!

Activity 12.2

▶ You will need your partner stripped to the waist for this activity. On your partner's chest, identify the following structures:

— Clavicle

— Coracoid process

— Manubrium sterni

— Sternal angle (of Louis)

— Sternoclavicular joint

— Acromioclavicular joint

— Body of sternum

— Xiphoid process

— 2nd intercostal space

— Costal margin

— Nipple

— Anterior axillary fold.

▶ Study the surface markings of the organs inside the chest. Note the extent of the pleural cavity superiorly approximately 3 cm above the clavicle (see also Ch. 6). Anteriorly and medially, the pleura on each side touch behind the sternal angle and move apart lower down. The left side moves away from the midline higher up than the right because of the heart. Note the surface markings of the pleura at the level of the 8th and 10th costal cartilages, and the 12th rib.

▶ Look at the surface markings of the lungs themselves on the anterior chest wall. Note that for the most part the extent of the lungs is the same as that of the pleura, but inferiorly the lungs do not extend downwards as far as the pleura into the lateral recesses. Note the surface markings of the lung fissures.

▶ Trace a line from the transverse process of the 4th thoracic vertebra to a point just medial to the 6th costochondral junction. This marks the course of the oblique fissure.

▶ On the right side, trace a horizontal line around your partner's chest from the level of the 4th costal cartilage until the line meets the line drawn for the oblique fissure. This marks the horizontal fissure, which is present only on the right side.

▶ Note the position of the trachea in the midline behind the suprasternal notch.

▶ Ask your partner to swallow, and note the movement of the thyroid cartilage during this manoeuvre. Note the level at which the trachea divides into the two main bronchi.

▶ Study the surface markings of the heart on the front of the chest. First of all, note whether your partner is tall or short, slender or stocky. The body build can markedly affect the position of the heart.

▶ Find the position of the middle of the clavicle, and trace a line vertically downwards from this point. This is called the mid-clavicular line, for obvious reasons. Note the point at which this line intersects the 5th intercostal space; the apex of the heart is normally found at this point.

▶ Place the pad of your middle finger at this point on your partner's chest and concentrate on palpating the cardiac impulse. The so-called 'apex beat' is defined as the most inferior and lateral point at which the cardiac impulse can be palpated, and in cases of cardiac enlargement it can be displaced outwards and downwards. Note:

— The position of the anterior axillary line, which is a vertical line drawn from the anterior axillary fold, formed by the pectoralis major muscle

— The mid-axillary line, which is a vertical line drawn midway between the anterior and posterior axillary folds.

▶ From the apex of the heart, draw a line horizontally to your partner's right until you reach the right side of the sternum. Now, continue your line vertically upwards along the right sternal edge until you meet the 2nd intercostal space. The line now travels horizontally to reach the 2nd intercostal space at the left sternal edge.

▶ Finally, join the apex to the point that you have just reached with a line which is slightly convex to the left. You have now traced the surface markings of the heart.

▶ Look at the surface markings of the valves of the heart. You will be listening to the sounds that the valves make at a later stage in this case study, but for now just note the position of the four heart valves:

— Mitral

— Tricuspid

— Aortic

— Pulmonary.

▶ Look at the surface markings of the great blood vessels entering and leaving the heart. Note:

— The position of the aorta, emerging from the aortic valve and travelling upwards and slightly to the right until it arches over the bifurcation of the pulmonary artery behind the sternal angle

— The position of the superior and inferior venae cavae just to the right of the sternum, and the point at which they enter the heart

— The origin of the major arteries from the arch of the aorta:

  – brachiocephalic

  – left common carotid

  – left subclavian.

Activity 12.3

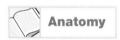 **Anatomy**

▶ Study the structure of the heart. You have already looked at the surface markings of the heart on the anterior chest wall. Now look at the relations of the heart within the thorax.

▶ Identify the four chambers of the heart, and how the great vessels enter and leave.

▶ Study the relationship of the phrenic and vagus nerves to the heart, and note particularly the left phrenic nerve lying on the left ventricle.

▶ Note the proximity of the two main bronchi, the oesophagus and the descending thoracic aorta to the posterior aspect of the heart, and note how the heart seems to be 'trapped' between the lungs on either side.

▶ Now study the vessels which supply the heart itself with blood. Note the emergence of the two coronary arteries from the aorta very close to the cusps of the aortic valve. Trace the course of the main coronary arteries and their branches. (It is possible to show the course of the arteries in the living person by means of injecting a radio-opaque dye into a coronary artery and taking X-rays as the dye travels down the vessels.) Note that the veins of the heart accompany the arteries, and drain into the coronary sinus.

Questions for discussion

- Why is the blood supply to the heart known as the 'coronary' circulation?
- Which areas of the heart are supplied by the
  - right coronary artery
  - left coronary artery
  - anterior interventricular artery
  - posterior interventricular artery
  - right marginal artery
  - left marginal artery?
- Are there any anastomoses between the main blood vessels of the heart? What would be their importance?

▶ Now look at the interior of the heart. Note:
  — The openings of the great vessels into and out of the four chambers
  — The arrangement of the muscle fibres in the right atrium
  — Note particularly the atrioventricular valves with the papillary muscles and the chordae tendinae which are attached to the cusps of the valves, and the pulmonary and aortic valves between the respective ventricle and the great vessels.

Question for discussion

- What might result from a rupture of the papillary muscles of one of the atrioventricular valves?

▶ Study the specialised conducting system of the heart. Note the position of the sinuatrial and atrioventricular nodes. Note also the bundle of His leading to the right and left bundles. The conducting system cannot be seen with the naked eye.

▶ Now look at the nerve supply to the heart. There are fibres from both sympathetic and parasympathetic divisions of the autonomic nervous system. Note particularly the position of the cardiac plexus in relation to the arch of the aorta, and the left and right coronary plexuses accompanying the respective coronary artery and supplying the respective atrium and ventricle.

Question for discussion

■ From which spinal segments does the sympathetic supply to the heart arise? Can you think of why this might be relevant to Mr Newman's symptoms?

Activity 12.4

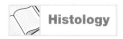 **Histology**

▶ Study the detailed structure of the tissues in the heart, starting with the structure of cardiac muscle cells.

▶ Look at a picture of cardiac muscle fibres in your textbook, and note that they form a sort of meshwork. The individual fibres are striated in a similar way to that of skeletal muscle, and the fibres contain actin and myosin filaments which can slide over each other during contraction. Note that the cardiac muscle cells are connected at their ends to other cells via an intercalated disc.

Questions for discussion

■ How is the arrangement of cardiac muscle cells different from that of skeletal muscle cells?

■ What other differences can you find between cardiac and skeletal muscle?

■ What is a syncytium? What do you think might be the functional significance of having the cardiac muscle cells arranged in a syncytium?

▶ Look at the structure of the specialised conducting system of the heart. Note:

— The structure of the cells in the sinuatrial and atrioventricular nodes, and the bundle of His

— That the nodal cells are narrower than ordinary cardiac muscle cells, but that the Purkinje cells of the bundles are generally wider

— Note particularly that the cells of the sinuatrial node are in contact with neighbouring myocardial cells, whereas those of the atrioventricular node and bundles are insulated from the rest of the myocardium by a connective tissue sheath.

Questions for discussion

■ What do you think are the functions of the cells of the conducting system?

■ What do you think might be the significance of the differences in fibre diameter of the various cells of the conduction system?

Activity 12.5

▶ You will need a mains water supply and a piece of tubing approximately 50 cm long that will fit over the water tap. Fit the tubing over the tap and turn on the water supply, fairly gently so as not to splash everything, but enough to give a steady stream.

▶ Grasp the middle of the tubing with one hand and rhythmically squeeze and relax your grip. Note what happens to the stream of water out of the tap. If you have performed this activity correctly, you should have found that the water stream reduced while you were squeezing, and increased while your grip was relaxed.

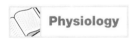 **Physiology**

▶ Now study the blood supply to the heart during the cardiac cycle. Note that the pattern of blood flow in the coronary arteries is similar to that which you have just demonstrated with the water supply.

Question for discussion

■ Why do you think that the coronary blood flow is greater in the diastolic phase of the cardiac cycle?

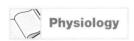 **Physiology**

▶ Study the control of coronary blood flow. Note that the demands of the heart for nutrition (mainly oxygen) form by far the major determinant of coronary blood flow, and that this is true even if the nerves to the heart have been destroyed. Note the different substances that have been proposed as vasodilators of the coronary vessels, and how they are released into the locality during increased activity of the cardiac muscle cells.

Questions for discussion

- How does an increase in the heart's demand for oxygen lead to a proportionate increase in coronary blood flow?
- How does stimulation of the autonomic nerves to the heart affect coronary blood flow?

Activity 12.6

▶ You will need a piece of thread, a felt-tip pen, two weights of about 100 g and 200 g, two weights of 1 kg and a piece of graph paper for this activity. Tie the 100 g weight to one end of the thread and the 200 g weight to the other end. Place the two heavier weights at the edge of a table and place the graph paper on the table near to these.

▶ Arrange the equipment as in Figure 12.1, with the felt-tip pen being held so that no movement of the thread occurs.

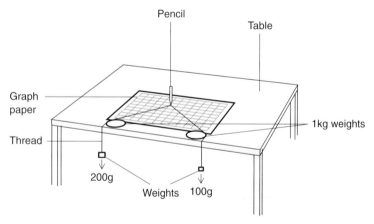

Fig. 12.1 Equipment for Activity 12.6.

▶ The pen will mark the initial point of departure onto the graph paper. From this point, mark along the lines of the thread towards the heavier weights, measuring 100 mm along the line going towards the 100 g weight and 200 mm along the line going towards the 200 g weight.

▶ Very gently release your pressure on the pen so that it can move under the influence of the two lighter weights, but still maintains enough pressure to write on the graph paper. The pen will trace out a wiggly line as it is driven by the thread. Draw a straight line on the graph paper to fit the first few centimetres of this line (see Fig. 12.2).

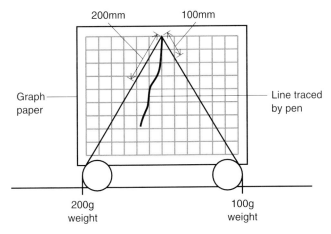

Fig. 12.2 The wavy line drawn by the pen.

▶ Now complete a parallelogram with the initial directions of the thread as the two sides from which to take the other two sides (see Fig. 12.3).

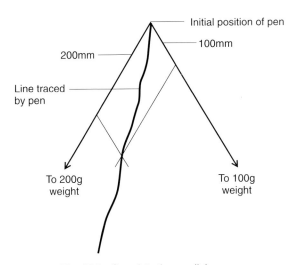

Fig. 12.3 Complete the parallelogram.

▶ Extend the straight line drawn from the initial direction of movement of the pen until it meets the far sides of the parallelogram that you have just drawn. How near does the line go to the far corner?

▶ You can repeat this experiment with different weights and different initial directions of the thread.

Questions for discussion

■ What do you understand by the term 'vector'?

■ What is the 'parallelogram of forces'? How does it relate to the experiment that you have just performed?

▶ Ask your local general practitioner if you can see an electrocardiographic trace. Alternatively, ask at your local hospital if you can observe an electrocardiogram being performed on a patient, or even on yourself if they are not too busy. If you cannot do either of these, take a look at Figure 12.4.

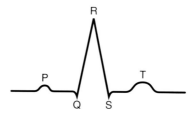

Fig. 12.4 Different types of waves on the electrocardiogram.

For this case, you will need to understand some basic ideas about how the electrocardiogram is formed. (There are further details regarding action potentials in nerve and muscle in Ch. 7.)

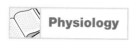 **Physiology**

▶ Study the major difference in the shape of the action potential of cardiac muscle compared to skeletal muscle or nerve. Note:

— That the action potential of cardiac muscle has a long 'plateau' phase and has a duration of around 300 ms

— The different shapes and durations of the action potentials from different areas of the heart, and in particular the diastolic depolarisation of the 'pacemaker' cells

— The sequence of electrical events that occurs during the course of a cardiac cycle

 — activation of the sinuatrial node

 — spread of excitation through the atria

- delay at the atrioventricular node
- fast conduction down the bundle of His
- spread of activity into the ventricular muscle.

The excitation of the cells of the heart is an electrical event, and so electrical currents flow into the surrounding tissues, and they may be detected by sensitive recording equipment such as an electrocardiograph. Electrical currents are vector quantities, and as such have direction as well as magnitude. The relevance to the electrocardiogram is that an electrode placed on the skin surface will detect whether the net direction of electrical current is flowing away from or towards it. By convention, current flowing towards an electrode results in an upwards (positive) deflection of the recording pen.

▶ Look at the directions of the cardiac vectors at different stages in the cardiac cycle, and try to relate these to the sequence of electrical events that occurs, and to what the deflection of an electrode placed in a particular position on the chest wall might be.

Questions for discussion

■ What electrical events in the heart cause the following waves on the electrocardiogram:
- P wave
- QRS complex
- T wave?

■ Given the shape of the cardiac action potential, how do you account for the shape of the electrocardiogram?

■ How does the autonomic nervous system affect the heart rate?

Having electrical activity in the heart is all very well, but it doesn't by itself pump the blood round the body. It is the mechanical activity of the heart muscle that does this. In fact, there is a condition known as electromechanical dissociation in which electrical signals continue to be recorded but there is no mechanical activity of the heart muscle. The patient is in cardiac arrest, and the outlook for this type of picture is very poor.

Activity 12.7

▶ You can construct very simply a crude model of the action of the heart. You will need a length of tubing about 50 cm long and 0.5 cm in diameter, two balloons and a tennis ball. Cut two small holes on opposite sides of the tennis ball, just smaller than the diameter of the tubing. Cut the tubing so that there is one length of about 10 cm and one of 40 cm. Cut the necks off the balloons, and pull them over one end of each of the pieces of tubing so that most of the neck is hanging free over the end (see Fig. 12.5).

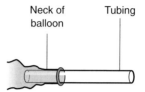

Fig. 12.5 To construct a model of the action of the heart fit balloons onto two lengths of tubing.

▶ Now thread the lengths of tubing into the holes in the tennis ball so that one piece of balloon is inside the ball and the other is on the outer end of the tubing (see Fig. 12.6).

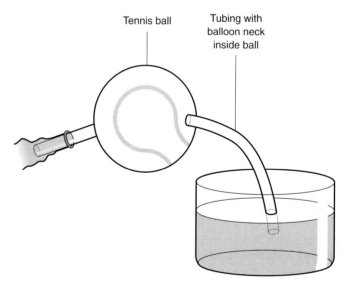

Fig. 12.6 Your model of 'the heart'.

▶ Dip the end of the tubing that is not covered by a piece of balloon into a beaker of water, and place the other end over a collection vessel. Now rhythmically squeeze the tennis ball and see what happens. If you have set things up correctly, you should find that water is drawn out of the beaker and eventually spurts out of the other end of the tubing.

▶ You can convert this into a 'circulation' by dipping the balloon-clad end of the tubing into the same beaker as the free end. You should find that the water continues to circulate around the system as long as you are squeezing the 'heart'.

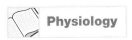 **Physiology**

▶ Now study how the heart actually pumps. Note that the action potential from the specialised conducting system spreads to the cardiac muscle and causes depolarisation of the membrane of the T-tubules and the sarcoplasmic reticulum. This causes calcium to enter the muscle sarcoplasm and initiate the interaction between the actin and myosin filaments that causes the contraction of the muscle. The whole process is known as excitation–contraction coupling.

Questions for discussion

- In which respects does the excitation–contraction coupling process of cardiac muscle differ from that of skeletal muscle?
- How would you explain the shape of the action potential of cardiac muscle?

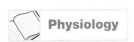 **Physiology**

▶ Study the events that occur in the cardiac cycle. Note that the cycle consists of diastole, a period of relaxation in which the heart fills with blood, and systole, which is when the heart muscle contracts and ejects blood into the rest of the circulation.

In most textbooks of physiology you will find a diagram detailing the pressure changes in the various chambers of the heart during the cardiac cycle, and the points at which the valves open and close. It is important that you become familiar with the concepts embodied in such a diagram, but it can appear quite daunting if you have not come across it before. You may find some assistance by going back to the model that you have made and going through the squeeze (systole) and relax (diastole) phases in slow motion.

You should note carefully the points at which the balloon 'valves' open and shut. If you imagine that the tennis ball is the ventricle, you should be able to determine which piece of tubing represents the atrium and which represents the outflow vessel (aorta or pulmonary artery). You may even be able to vary some of the conditions that occur under 'physiological' conditions. For example, you could vary the 'heart rate' by varying the frequency of squeeze, and the 'stroke volume' may be altered by varying the degree of squeeze at each systole. (NB: you will need your model again for Activity 12.10.)

Questions for discussion

- What is the relationship between the waves on the electrocardiogram and the mechanical events in the cardiac cycle?
- During the phases of the cardiac cycle what happens in
    - isovolumic relaxation
    - rapid ventricular filling
    - isovolumic contraction
    - ejection?
- Why are the pressures recorded in the right ventricle during the cardiac cycle much smaller than those recorded in the left ventricle?

You should now be in a position to describe what happens in a cardiac cycle. Now you need to study how the heart is controlled. First, you can do a little physical and mental limbering up.

Activity 12.8

- ▶ Rest for a few minutes and take your pulse rate (you could do this activity with a partner, but it isn't necessary).
- ▶ Now run on the spot for 5 minutes. Take your pulse rate at 1-minute intervals after you have stopped running and plot the results on a graph. Continue your recording until the pulse rate is back to the resting level. You should find that the heart rate increases substantially during the exercise, and gradually returns to the resting level in a few minutes after the exercise is stopped.

Question for discussion

- Can you devise an experiment to investigate how fitness affects the rate at which the heart rate returns to the resting level after exercise?

▶ Repeat the exercise, but now feel the strength of the heart beat as you are exercising. Can you feel that there is greater force of pumping action?

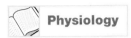
Physiology

▶ Now study the control of the pumping action of the heart. Note the two main factors:

— Intrinsic regulation – Starling's 'law of the heart'

— Extrinsic regulation – autonomic nervous system.

If you think about the circulation of blood through the heart, you will realise that, over a period of time, the amount of blood that is ejected from the heart must be equal to the amount of blood that enters the heart. Starling's law explains in physiological terms why this is so.

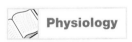
Physiology

▶ If you study the mechanics of skeletal muscle, you will come across a 'length–tension curve', which expresses the relationship between the initial length of a muscle fibre and the tension that the fibre produces during its contraction. A similar relationship holds for cardiac muscle.

Questions for discussion

■ How can you explain Starling's law of the heart on the basis of the length–tension curve?

■ How can you explain the length–tension curve in terms of the interaction of actin and myosin filaments in the muscle cell?

Examination 1

On examination, Mr Newman looked reasonably well, and was not breathless or in obvious pain at rest. There was no evidence of anaemia, jaundice, cyanosis or clubbing of the fingers (see Ch. 11 for more information on clubbing of the fingers). The pulse rate was 70 per minute and regular, but when you felt the pulse it appeared to rise and fall slowly. Blood pressure was 110/80 mmHg. Palpation of the chest revealed that the heart apex beat was slightly displaced to the 6th intercostal space in the anterior axillary line, and the left ventricular impulse was very forceful. Auscultation of the heart showed that there was a mid-systolic murmur heard best in the 2nd intercostal space on the right, and the murmur could be heard right up into the neck. Detailed examination of the musculoskeletal system showed a lot of tightness and tenderness in the trapezius muscles, which seemed to be contracted most of the time so that Mr Newman's shoulders always had a hunched appearance. The thoracic spine showed restriction to movement at T2–T4, and at these levels there was excess moisture on the skin and a feeling of sponginess on palpation of the skin.

Questions for discussion

- What is a heart murmur?
- What is the difference between a systolic and a diastolic murmur?
- What causes can you think of for Mr Newman's murmur?
- Why do you think that Mr Newman's apex beat was displaced to the left?
- What relevance do you think the past history of rheumatic fever has to Mr Newman's present condition?
- What do you think is the significance of Mr Newman's forceful left ventricular impulse?
- What do you think is the significance of Mr Newman's abnormal pulse?
- How might you account for the findings in the thoracic spine?
- Which further investigations do you think might be helpful for Mr Newman?

Activity 12.9

 Clinical examination

▶ You will need a stethoscope for this activity, and your partner should be stripped to the waist. But first, study the examination of the heart.

You will note that there are general features of the examination (such as examination of the peripheral pulses, examination for anaemia and cyanosis, and assessment of peripheral oedema) that enable you to make a complete assessment of cardiac function. Some of these are discussed in other chapters (e.g. Ch. 2 for activities on peripheral oedema, and Chs 8 and 10 for activities on anaemia). For this case, you should concentrate on the examination of the heart sounds, and on assessing the rate and force of contraction of the heart. Your textbook will tell you where to put the stethoscope to best hear the heart sounds emanating from the different heart valves.

▶ First, feel for your partner's apex beat, as in Activity 12.2. This time, as well as just noting the position of the impulse, you should assess its forcefulness and the rate and rhythm of the heart beat.

▶ Now listen to your partner's chest in the following places, and carefully note the sounds that you hear at the:

— Apex

— 2nd intercostal space, just to the right of the sternum

— 2nd intercostal space, just to the left of the sternum

— 5th intercostal space, at the left sternal edge.

Generally, heart sounds are heard better on thinner people.

Questions for discussion

■ Why are the heart sounds from the different valves heard best at the places indicated?

■ What do you think is the relationship between the heart sounds that you hear and the phases of the cardiac cycle?

■ Try to work out the significance of the mid-systolic murmur heard in Mr Newman.

Examination 2

Mr Newman had an electrocardiogram, which showed left ventricular hypertrophy, and a chest X-ray, which showed some enlargement of the left ventricle. The lateral film showed a calcified aortic valve.

Echocardiography showed thickening of the left ventricular wall and calcification of the aortic valve.

Mr Newman was then sent to the regional cardiac centre for cardiac catheterisation. This showed a reduced gradient of pressure across the aortic valve. Coronary angiography was essentially normal.

Questions for discussion

- Why should Mr Newman's heart be enlarged?
- What is the significance of the calcified aortic valve?
- What are the electrocardiographic criteria for left ventricular hypertrophy?
- What is the significance of the reduced pressure gradient across the aortic valve?
- What is the diagnosis?

Activity 12.10

▶ For this activity you will need the tennis ball, tubing and balloon model of the heart and circulation that you used in Activity 12.7. Vary the resistance to flow offered by the 'aortic' valve (i.e. the piece of balloon neck that is attached to the outflow from the 'ventricle'). You can do this by varying the amount of balloon that protrudes from the end of the tubing or by attaching an adjustable clip to the outflow tubing.

▶ Repeat the squeeze/relax cycle with varying amounts of restriction of the outflow tube, and note any difference in the flow of water through the outflow (see also Ch. 3 for more information on resistance to flow). If you have the protruding balloon above the level of water in the beaker, you will be able to see the outflow, and you can note how forcefully the water is ejected.

Questions for discussion

- What happens to the water jet as you vary the outflow resistance?
- If you had a means of measuring the water pressure on either side of the outflow valve, what do you think would happen to the

drop in pressure across the valve if the outflow resistance were increased?

■ What relevance do you think that this experiment has to Mr Newman's cardiac catheterisation findings?

▶ Look back at Activity 1.12. Note that a musical sound is heard when there is air flow through a narrowed orifice.

▶ Using your model of the heart, get your partner to squeeze the neck of the balloon acting as the outflow valve while you continue to squeeze the tennis ball 'ventricle'. Do you get a noise as the water is forced through the narrowed exit?

▶ Vary the force with which you squeeze the tennis ball and note whether this makes any difference to the sound that you hear.

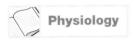

Physiology

▶ Now study again the diagram that shows the pressures in the various chambers of the heart during the cardiac cycle. Similar patterns hold for both right and left sides of the heart except that the pressures in the left side are much higher, so if the diagram in your textbook shows pressures in the right side, just imagine that it is the left side and adjust the numbers.

Questions for discussion

■ Which heart valve on the left side is normally open in systole? Is it open throughout the whole of systole?

■ How does the left ventricle compensate for an increased resistance through the aortic valve? What relevance does this have to the electrocardiographic, X-ray and echocardiographic findings on Mr Newman?

You have had a lot of anatomy and physiology to study for this case. Perhaps it is time to turn to a bit of psychology and to examine briefly the relationship between stress and illness. You will remember from the initial history that Mr Newman was working under pressure and may even have been feeling that he had to live up to his illustrious namesake.

Activity 12.11

▶ Think about your own situation. If you have ever had to take

an examination, go for an important job interview, speak up
or play an instrument in front of an audience, try to remember
what feelings you had. Did you get 'butterflies' in your
stomach?

▶ Think also about any time you may have had an unexpected
fright, such as a loud noise or coming upon someone
unexpectedly. Did your pulse start to race, and did you feel
'palpitations' as the heart started to beat more forcefully?

Question for discussion

■ What mechanisms can you think of that might produce the
cardiovascular effects seen during stress?

There is quite a lot of research work into the relationship
between psychosocial factors and diseases. Most of this work
tends to use techniques of epidemiology, i.e. large populations
are studied in an attempt to identify particular psychosocial
factors which are associated with a higher risk of developing
certain diseases.

Questions for discussion

■ What value do you think the epidemiological approach has for the
study of the relationship between stress and illness?

■ Can you think of any limitations of the approach when dealing with
individual patients such as Mr Newman?

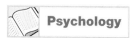 **Psychology**

▶ Study how chronic stress might influence the production of
heart disease. Note that there are a number of theories, but
most of them propose that personality characteristics or life
situations result in an elevated level of adrenaline in the
blood. This would have various effects on the cardiovascular
system.

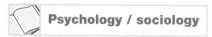 **Psychology / sociology**

▶ Study the theory that 'life events' such as bereavement or loss
of a job influence the development of disease. Note that
positive as well as negative events may have an effect.

However, a complicating factor in the interpretation of this type of theory is that different people will vary in their response to a particular life event. In other words, it seems to be the meaning of the event for the individual, together with the person's ability to cope with the situation, that determines susceptibility to stress-induced illness.

Questions for discussion

- What effects can you think of that increased adrenaline levels would have on:
  - blood clotting
  - blood cholesterol levels
  - arterial blood pressure
  - the work of the heart?
- What is a 'Type A' personality? Do you think that Mr Newman has such a personality?
- What relevance do you think that Mr Newman's feelings of being stressed have to the generation of his symptoms?
- How would you go about investigating the relationship between 'Type A' personality and heart disease?

Discussion

One of the main considerations for this case is that it is relatively easy to diagnose ischaemic heart disease, but perhaps the lesson which you should take home is that there may be a structural abnormality underlying the cardiac ischaemia. The vast majority of patients with angina pectoris have atherosclerotic narrowing of the coronary arteries, but occasionally other causes such as anaemia and aortic stenosis may give rise to angina. With all causes of angina, the underlying pathophysiology is an inability of the body to supply enough oxygen to keep up with the demand of the heart. Severe anaemia results in a reduction of the oxygen-carrying capacity of the blood, and it is easy to see how this might cause angina.

Aortic stenosis is rather uncommon nowadays because of the decline in the incidence of rheumatic fever. Nevertheless, it is important for you to think of this diagnosis when presented with a patient with features of ischaemic heart disease. (It is also useful for you to study the mechanical events of the cardiac cycle in general.) Aortic stenosis may arise as a result of a bicuspid aortic valve (where the aortic valve has two cusps instead of the usual three) or from senile calcification invading the cusps.

The reaction of the left ventricle to the increased resistance to the outflow of blood is to increase its muscle mass in order to create a higher pressure to force the blood out. The end-diastolic pressure in the left ventricle is thus high. This has two main results:

— The increased muscle mass has a higher demand for oxygen

— The perfusion of the coronary arteries is reduced.

Angina may thus occur without atheroma of the coronary arteries. Eventually, the left ventricle may not be able to cope with the increased demands, resulting in the features of left ventricular failure. The heart may not be able to increase its cardiac output during exercise, and this may lead to syncope on exertion or even to sudden death.

The main physical signs of aortic stenosis are:

— A slow-rising pulse

— A forceful left ventricular impulse

— An ejection systolic murmur, heard best at the left upper sternal edge and radiating into the neck.

An ejection systolic murmur occurs only when blood is being forced through the narrowed valve during systole. If you refer back to the diagram of pressures in the heart chambers during the cardiac cycle, you will note that the ejection phase does not take up the whole of systole. Thus you will hear heart sounds on either side of the murmur.

Investigation of suspected aortic valve stenosis will include electrocardiography to confirm the left ventricular hypertrophy. It may also show conduction blocks due to invasion of the conducting system by the calcium from the valve. Chest X-ray may show a calcified aortic valve, and a large left ventricle if it is failing. Echocardiography may show the valve orifice and the reduced movement of the valve. Cardiac catheterisation will show a reduced pressure gradient across the aortic valve, and can also be used to analyse left ventricular function.

Treatment of aortic stenosis is mainly surgical, with replacement of the affected valve. If there is no heart failure, the results are quite good.

There is little that the manual therapist can do to relieve the situation. The pathological process will not be reversed by treatment of either the soft tissues or the spinal or peripheral joints, although you may be able to reduce Mr Newman's oxygen demand a little by measures to reduce his stress level. The main point is to recognise the possibility of the condition and refer the patient to a medical practitioner for further management.

FURTHER READING

Mangion J R, Tighe D A 1995 Aortic valvular disease in adults. A potentially lethal clinical problem. Postgraduate Medicine 98: 127–135

Pellikka P A, Nishimura R A, Bailey K R, Tajik A 1990 The natural history of adults with asymptomatic haemodynamically significant aortic stenosis. Journal of the American College of Cardiologists 15: 1018–1020

Mrs Catherine Kendall

Study objectives

After studying this case with its associated activities and questions, you should have a reasonable knowledge of the following areas:

1. Surface anatomy of structures in the lumbar area
2. Surface markings of organs on the posterior abdominal wall
3. Anatomical relations of the kidneys
4. Blood and nerve supply to the kidneys
5. Structure of lumbar vertebrae
6. Arrangement of the ligaments of the lumbar vertebral column
7. Structure of intervertebral discs
8. Attachments, actions, blood and nerve supply of muscles acting on the lumbar spine
9. Blood supply of the spine and spinal cord
10. Nerve supply of the lumbar vertebrae
11. Palpating the soft tissues in the lumbar area
12. Testing the gross movements of the lumbar spine
13. Biomechanics of movement of the lumbar spine
14. Causes of low back pain
15. Histology of the nephron
16. Arrangement of the blood supply to the nephron
17. Mechanisms by which the kidneys eliminate waste products
18. General features of negative feedback mechanisms
19. Regulation of the level of calcium in the blood
20. Histology of parathyroid glands
21. Actions of parathyroid hormone and calcitonin
22. Causes of hypercalcaemia
23. Clinical features of hypercalcaemia
24. Examination of a plain abdominal X-ray film

25. Examination of an intravenous urogram
26. Types of kidney stones
27. Clinical features of kidney stones.

Background

Mrs Catherine Kendall, a 55-year-old typist, felt that she had enjoyed pretty good health throughout her life. She was not someone who liked to trouble the doctor about minor complaints, so when she developed some discomfort in the back, she felt that she would be better off going directly to a private therapist who would be able to sort out the problem.

When you questioned her further regarding the discomfort, Mrs Kendall told you that it was a dull ache located mainly in the left loin area. The pain did not radiate anywhere, and she did not feel generally unwell, apart from a general lack of energy over the previous few months.

Questions for discussion

- What other questions would you ask Mrs Kendall about her pain?

- Are there any other questions that you think are relevant to ask Mrs Kendall at this stage?

On further questioning, Mrs Kendall told you that there were no particular factors which worsened or relieved the discomfort, and that since the pain had come on only a few days previously, it was difficult to tell whether it was getting worse or better. She did report that she had experienced the occasional 'tummy ache' in the recent past, associated with being off her food and with vomiting but without loss of weight. Her bowels were usually a bit 'bunged up' as she put it, but there was no pain or blood on passing her motions. She had experienced some minor problems with urination in that she had noticed passing some gravelly material, but she did not feel that she was unduly thirsty and she did not have an increased frequency of urination.

Questions for discussion

■ What are your thoughts concerning the cause of Mrs Kendall's discomfort?

■ To which points in the physical examination would you pay special attention?

Activity 13.1

▶ You will need to have your partner undressed to his underpants for this activity. On your partner's back, identify the following structures:

— Iliac crest

— Posterior superior iliac spine (PSIS)

— 12th rib

— Spine of 12th thoracic vertebra

— Spines of lumbar vertebrae

— Transverse processes of lumbar vertebrae.

▶ Now draw a line between the iliac crests. This is called the intercristal line, and should pass between the spines of the 3rd and 4th lumbar vertebrae.

Questions for discussion

■ At which vertebral level does the spinal cord end? What difference in this level is there between an adult and a child?

■ What is a lumbar puncture?

■ Where is the needle placed when performing a lumbar puncture?

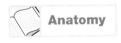 **Anatomy**

▶ Study the surface markings of the organs near to the posterior abdominal wall. The main organs that you will find in this exercise are the kidneys, adrenal glands and the spleen.

▶ Draw a vertical line from the top of the iliac crest, and another along the tips of the transverse processes of the lumbar vertebrae. Now draw horizontal lines at the level of the spinous process of the 12th thoracic and 3rd lumbar vertebrae. You will be left with a box on each side, which roughly delineates the boundaries of the kidneys.

▶ Draw a kidney bean shape in each box, with the indentation (hilus) facing medially and slightly downwards. You should find that the hilus is approximately in the transpyloric plane, which is a horizontal line at the level of the lower border of the 1st lumbar vertebra.

▶ Observe the difference in levels between the right and left kidneys. Why should this be so? Note also the overlap of the diaphragmatic pleura, and consider the structures that would be affected by trauma to the kidney area.

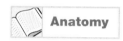 **Anatomy**

▶ Study the other relationships of the kidneys. Note particularly the close proximity to the diaphragm, lower ribs, liver, spleen, pancreas, stomach, duodenum, small and large intestines, aorta and inferior vena cava, and also to the muscles on the posterior abdominal wall (psoas major, quadratus lumborum, transversus abdominis). Note also the suprarenal (adrenal) glands which lie attached to the superior pole of each kidney. Each gland is approximately 1 cm × 3 cm × 5 cm in size, and is roughly pyramid shaped.

▶ Look at the blood supply to the kidneys. Note:

— The origin of the renal artery from the aorta, and how it divides into several branches before entering the substance of the kidney at the hilus

— The renal vein arising from the hilus and passing to the inferior vena cava

— The lymphatic vessels arising from the hilus and draining into the aortic lymph nodes.

▶ Study the pelvis of the ureter as it widens into the kidney hilus, and note the major and minor calyces of the kidney as they project into the pelvis.

▶ Study the nerve supply of the kidney. First of all, study the coeliac plexus, which is the largest of the sympathetic plexuses. It is located at the thoracolumbar junction and surrounds the coeliac artery and the root of the superior mesenteric artery.

▶ Look at the greater and lesser splanchnic nerves, which supply the plexus, and note that the phrenic and vagus nerves give some nerve fibres to the plexus.

▶ Note the secondary plexuses arising from the coeliac plexus, and in particular the renal plexus. This receives nerve fibres from other plexuses and nerves in addition to the supply from the coeliac plexus, namely the splanchnic nerves from T12 and L1, the aortic plexus and the aorticorenal ganglion. The nerves from the renal plexus surround the renal artery to supply the vessels of the renal glomeruli and tubules.

Questions for discussion

■ What are the functions of the nerve supply to the kidney?

■ How do you think your knowledge of the nerve supply to the kidney is relevant to Mrs Kendall's pain?

Activity 13.2

▶ You will again need your partner stripped to his underpants for this activity. Ask your partner to stand with his back to you with his feet approximately 15 cm apart and the weight evenly distributed between the legs. Observe the shape of your partner's spine, paying particular attention in this case study to the lumbar region.

▶ Look at your partner's lumbar spine from the front, sides and back. Note the symmetry of the spine when viewed from the front and back, and note the curve which should be convex anteriorly when you view him from the side. This is the lumbar lordosis.

▶ While looking at your partner from the back, ask him to bend his right knee slightly, and take the weight of his body mainly on the left leg. Note how the whole spine shifts to the right, but note particularly that the lumbar spine shows a curve which is concave towards the left, and that the left hip is higher than the right.

Questions for discussion

■ Why does your partner not fall over when he stands with his weight mainly on one leg?

■ How does the rest of the vertebral column compensate for the lateral curvature of the lumbar spine?

Activity 13.3

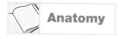 **Anatomy**

▶ You are going to palpate the soft tissues in your partner's back. It is very useful to have a mental picture of the structures that you are feeling as you progress to various layers, so it might be helpful at this stage to revise the structure of the skin, subcutaneous tissues (including connective tissue, fat and fascia) and underlying muscles, tendons and ligaments. You will need to develop a methodical approach to soft tissue palpation, and to practise repeatedly in order to develop your skills.

Questions for discussion

- Which sensory endings in your skin are used to send information about the following modalities in your partner:
  - touch
  - temperature?
- Why is it necessary to rest your fingers during a palpatory session in order to ensure maximum sensitivity?

▶ Have your partner lie prone on an examination couch or on the floor. First of all, you should observe the skin on your partner's back. Note whether the area is pale or red, and whether there are areas of swelling. Note also any scars, bruises, cuts or grazes which might indicate trauma. If there are any abnormal areas, it will be useful to concentrate on these to compare them with the normal areas.

▶ Next, determine which area of your hand is most sensitive to temperature change. You can do this by taking two beakers of water at slightly different temperatures and touching each one alternately with the different parts of your hand. Very often it is the back of the fingers, but it could be the side of the hand, the fingertips or even the wrist. Palpate your partner's skin lightly so as not to induce vasodilatation, and compare different areas of the back for temperature differences. You could extend the activity to comparing the temperature at the same area in several people.

▶ Now slide your fingertips lightly down your partner's back in a smooth continuous movement, and note any difference in resistance to the movement of your fingers. This resistance is called 'skin drag', and may be due to a fine film of moisture on the skin surface.

Questions for discussion

■ Which nerves cause the skin to become moist?

■ What might be the significance of finding an area of increased skin drag?

▶ Stroke the skin of your partner's back with the tips of your fingers on either side of the spine at the same time. Use a firm pressure, sufficient to make the skin turn white (blanch) under the finger but not sufficient to cause pain. Note how long it takes for the skin colour to return to normal, comparing each side. Compare the degree of redness (erythema) on either side of the spine.

▶ Repeat the procedure using a ruler and a much firmer pressure while you stroke the skin on your partner's back. Note the response of the skin to this.

▶ Feel how rough or smooth the skin is on your partner's back.

▶ Compare the skin of the back with that in other areas of the body.

▶ Press gently on the skin and note whether it is 'springy' or whether it has a 'doughy' feel to it.

▶ Take an overripe pear and push your finger into it. You should find that it is easy to indent it, and that the indentation stays after you release the pressure. The same thing happens when there is oedema, which is excess fluid in the tissues. When you are pressing into the pear, note the 'dead' feel.

▶ If you know someone who suffers from oedema of the legs, ask if you may gently press the area of oedema. You should experience the same 'dead' feeling.

▶ Repeat the experiment with a lump of freshly prepared dough. You should find that the dough has quite a different feel, with a springiness that is not there in the pear. In this sense, the dough feels more 'alive' than the pear (see also Ch. 2 for more activities on oedema).

▶ Take a fold of skin between your finger and thumb, and then let it go. Note how quickly it returns to its original shape.

Questions for discussion

- What is the 'triple response'?
- What might cause localised oedema in the skin overlying the lumbar spine?

Activity 13.4

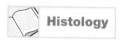 **Histology**

▶ When you have practised palpating the superficial layers of the skin, you should concentrate your efforts on the deeper layers, such as subcutaneous tissue, muscle and tendon. Again, it may be helpful to review the histology of these tissues to fix in your mind the structures that you are palpating.

▶ You can test your palpatory sensitivity in several ways, but the following is an easy method. You will need a telephone directory, or other thick book, and a single strand of hair. Place the hair inside the back cover of the directory and close it, so that the hair is under the pages. Run the tips of your fingers across the front of the directory to try to feel where the hair is. Concentrate all of your thoughts on the tip of the fingers.

▶ If you cannot feel the hair, open the directory a few pages and repeat the palpation.

▶ Repeat this until you can definitely sense the hair. Note the number of pages between your fingers and the hair.

▶ Keep practising this, and you should find that the number of pages between your fingertips and the hair increases.

▶ Get your partner to test your sensitivity by placing the hair somewhere on the page while you are not looking; try to determine where it is.

Palpating over bone will give you an idea of the feel of skin and subcutaneous tissue.

▶ Palpate over the medial and lateral malleoli, and note the quality of the tissues, especially their springiness and turgor.

▶ Place your thumb and first finger about 1 cm apart on your partner's back. Gently pull the tips of the digits apart until the 'slack' is taken up.

▶ Determine the resistance to further gentle stretching, and compare several different areas of skin.

▶ Palpate an area where there are superficial veins, such as the front of the elbow or forearm, and note the springiness of the veins. Compare this with the feel of an artery such as the radial or brachial.

▶ You can eliminate the pulsation of the radial artery by tying a tourniquet or blood pressure cuff around the upper arm (but don't leave the tourniquet on for more than a minute or so). This should also make the veins more prominent. Compare the feel of the artery and vein with the tourniquet applied.

▶ With your partner prone, press more deeply into his back until you feel the muscle fibres. Note the tone of the paraspinal muscles.

▶ Ask your partner to lift his knees 3 cm off the couch while you palpate the contraction of his paraspinal muscles. Palpate the relaxation of the muscles as your partner relaxes.

▶ Repeat the contraction–relaxation cycle with a weight placed on your partner's legs so that it is not possible for him to lift them off the couch. Ask him to try his hardest to lift his legs, and compare the contraction under these circumstances (isometric) with that in the previous conditions.

In some people, particularly those who worry a lot, muscles maintain their contraction even though there is no need for it. Have you ever noticed the furrowed brow or the elevated shoulders of a person who is worrying about something? If this contraction is maintained, the muscle may become chronically contracted and fibrous changes may occur. This makes the muscle feel like a length of rope or string which can be rolled under the fingers.

Questions for discussion

■ What factors determine skin resistance?

■ What physiological changes might occur in a muscle when it is chronically contracted?

Activity 13.5

▶ Kneel behind your standing partner and place your right hand on his right iliac crest and your left hand on his left iliac crest. Are they in the same horizontal plane or is one higher than the other?

Question for discussion

■ What causes are there for a discrepancy in the heights of the iliac crests?

▶ Place your thumb on your partner's posterior superior iliac spine on the respective side, and monitor the movement of your thumbs as you instruct your partner to perform the following movements:
— Slowly bend forwards as if to touch his toes, with his knees locked in extension
— Slowly bend backwards from the waist
— Slowly slide each hand in turn down the side of the ipsilateral leg, keeping the leg straight and without forward or backward bending
— Slowly turn his body to each side in turn, from the waist, keeping the knees extended and not moving the feet.

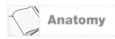 **Anatomy**

▶ Study the structure of a lumbar vertebra. Note:
— The shape of the body
— The plane of the laminae
— The shape and direction of the transverse processes
— The shape and direction of the spinous processes
— The attachments of the transverse processes
— The pedicles, forming the superior and inferior limits of the intervertebral foramen
— The structure and plane of the superior articular process
— The structure and plane of the inferior articular process
— The shape of the vertebral foramen.

▶ Observe how the inferior articular process of one lumbar vertebra fits into the superior articular process of the vertebra below it.

▶ Compare the arrangement of the articular surfaces in the lumbar and thoracic regions of the spine.

Questions for discussion

■ How does the arrangement of the articular processes limit the movement of the lumbar spine?

■ At which vertebral level does a functional transition from thoracic to lumbar regions occur? What movements are allowed at this transitional level?

Activity 13.6

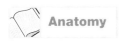 **Anatomy**

▶ Study the ligaments of the lumbar vertebral column. Note:

— The anterior and posterior longitudinal ligaments running from the occiput to the sacrum, and in particular their attachments to the intervertebral discs

— The different layers of the anterior ligament, with the most superficial fibres extending over several vertebrae while the deepest extend only from one vertebra to the next

— That the posterior longitudinal ligament does not attach to the middle of the vertebral bodies, and there is a space between it and the posterior surface of the vertebrae in which a venous plexus runs

— The ligamenta flava attached to the laminae, and nearly fusing in the midline to close off the vertebral canal; they are made of elastic tissue and are at their thickest in the lumbar region of the spine

— The capsular ligaments between the articular processes

— The supraspinous ligament, a strong fibrous cord which joins the apices of the vertebral spines, the thin interspinous ligament and the intertransverse ligaments, which are thin in the lumbar region.

Questions for discussion

■ What do you think are the functions of the ligaments in the lumbar spine?

■ How are the differences in movements of the different areas of the spine reflected in the different structure of the ligaments in each region?

■ During side-bending, why do the vertebrae rotate to the opposite side of the concavity of the side-bending?

Activity 13.7

▶ You will need some thin-walled rubber tubing approximately 2 cm in diameter and 1 cm in length, some unmade jelly and two pieces of dowelling (or cork) about 2 cm in diameter for this activity. Make up the jelly with less than the stated amount of water so that it is quite thick, putting the piece of rubber tubing into the container so that the jelly fills the tubing. When the jelly has set, take out the piece of tubing and remove excess jelly from around the tubing. The result should look something like Figure 13.1.

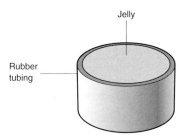

Fig. 13.1 A model of an intervertebral disc.

▶ Now glue the two pieces of dowelling to the top and bottom of the cylinder. You now have a very simple model of a functional unit of the spine (see Fig. 13.2), with the dowelling representing the vertebrae and the tubing plus jelly representing the intervertebral disc. (If you have more tubing and jelly, you can repeat the process to form a 'spine'.)

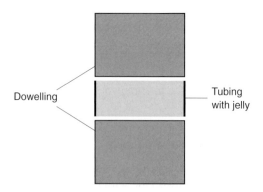

Fig. 13.2 A simple model of a functional unit of the spine.

▶ Make the model a little more complex by putting a staple into each of the pieces of dowelling to represent the vertebral arches of the upper and lower vertebrae; you could even solder on a short piece of metal to the apex of the staple to represent the spinous process. Don't get too carried away though, because you will lose the main point, which is the study of the intervertebral disc.

For ease of description, I will call the side of the dowelling in which the staples are inserted the 'posterior' aspect, since the vertebral arch is posterior to the body.

▶ Press the two staples apart to represent 'flexion' of the spine. Note how the tubing is stretched posteriorly and relaxed anteriorly. The tubing is thus wedge-shaped.

▶ Now let go of the staples. The vertebral unit should spring back to its original position.

▶ Repeat the experiment with extension and side-bending.

▶ Press the pieces of dowelling towards each other to represent the pressure of weight-bearing or load-bearing, and pull them apart gently to illustrate the effect of traction. Note the shape of the tubing in each case.

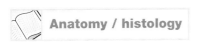 **Anatomy / histology**

▶ Study the structure and function of the intervertebral disc. Note:

— The structure of the nucleus pulposus and the annulus fibrosus

— That the nucleus contains no blood vessels or nerves, and so is not believed to be the site of pain

— The concentric fibres which make up the annulus, and the varying direction of the fibres which make up each layer

— That the nucleus is roughly spherical, and is held under pressure so that it tends to bulge if the annulus is cut.

Questions for discussion

■ If there were no bony, muscular or ligamentous structures to limit the movement between vertebrae, what movements would be allowed between the adjacent vertebral bodies?

- How does standing cause increased lateral force on the annulus?
- Why is a person taller in the morning than in the evening?
- How does the thickness of the disc vary with the region of the spine?
- Why is the nucleus not exactly at the centre of the disc?
- How is the disc innervated?

Activity 13.8

▶ Ask your partner to strip to the waist and stand erect. Feel the muscles on the posterior aspect of the spine.

▶ Ask your partner to slightly extend his back (i.e. lean backwards). You should note that the muscles relax.

▶ Now ask him to slowly flex his trunk while you continue to feel the muscles. You should find that as your partner flexes slightly beyond the upright, the posterior trunk muscles spring into action.

▶ Ask your partner to lie supine on an examination couch. Put one hand on the muscles of the anterior abdominal wall. Feel them while your partner is relaxed.

▶ Now ask him to try to lift both legs off the couch while you resist the movement with your other hand. Note the contraction of the muscles. You could also ask your partner to perform sit-ups.

▶ Ask your partner to lie prone, and feel the posterior trunk muscles. Ask him to lift his shoulders off the couch while you continue to feel the muscles. They should contract strongly.

▶ Study the muscles of the trunk. Note the attachments, actions, blood supply and nerve supply of the following muscles:
— Posterior muscles
  - transversospinalis
  - longissimus
  - iliocostalis
  - spinalis
  - serratus posterior inferior
  - latissimus dorsi
— Lateral muscles
  - quadratus lumborum
  - psoas

— Anterior muscles
  – transversus abdominis
  – obliquus internus abdominis
  – obliquus externus abdominis
  – rectus abdominis.

▶ Note that although the posterior muscles of the trunk act to extend the trunk, they do not straighten it. Indeed, their action tends to increase the curvature of the lumbar spine, in a similar manner to a bowstring.

▶ Note the actions of the lateral muscles in side-bending the trunk, and in particular the effect of the psoas muscle in increasing the lumbar lordosis and in rotating the trunk to the opposite side.

▶ Note the action of the muscles of the anterior abdominal wall forming a sort of 'corset' around the abdomen.

Questions for discussion

■ Which muscles are important in determining the curve of the waist?

■ How do the muscles of the anterior abdominal wall act to protect the spine when lifting a weight?

■ What action do the posterior muscles of the trunk have on the anteroposterior curvature of the thoracic spine?

■ Why is it better to lift weights with the trunk vertical rather than flexed?

Activity 13.9

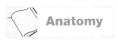 Anatomy

▶ Study the blood supply of the spine and spinal cord in the lumbar region. Note the lumbar arteries branching from the back of the aorta and in turn giving off a posterior ramus which supplies the muscles and skin of the back as well as the vertebrae and contents of the vertebral canal (the latter via the spinal branch). The spinal branch of the 1st lumbar artery also supplies the lower portion of the spinal cord.

▶ Study the anatomy of the spinal arteries, and in particular the anterior and posterior radicular arteries and the anterior and posterior spinal arteries.

Questions for discussion

- Which spinal tracts are damaged if the anterior spinal artery is occluded? What might be the clinical presentation of such a process?

▶ Study the complicated arrangement of veins draining blood from the vertebral column. Note:
  — The external and internal venous plexuses
  — The absence of valves and the free anastomoses in this system of veins
  — The basivertebral veins connecting the internal and external vertebral venous plexuses
  — The drainage of the venous system into the lumbar veins and also eventually into the vertebral veins.

Questions for discussion

- What happens to the vertebral venous flow when you perform a Valsalva manoeuvre?
- Why is the vertebral venous system important in the spread of malignant tumours?

Activity 13.10

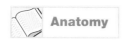 **Anatomy**

▶ Study the nerve supply to the vertebrae and associated structures. Note the anterior and posterior primary divisions of the nerve root. Note particularly the course of the recurrent meningeal nerve as it enters the grey matter. It contains fibres from the sympathetic ganglia, and supplies the anterior and posterior longitudinal ligaments, the dura of the nerve roots and the outer layer of the annulus fibrosus of the intervertebral disc.

Questions for discussion

- What other tissues in the vertebral functional unit are potential sites of pain production?
- Which viscera are innervated by nerves arising from the lumbar vertebrae? For each organ, describe the area of referred pain.

Examination

On physical examination, Mrs Kendall had very few abnormal physical signs that you could easily relate to her presentation. Her blood pressure was moderately elevated at 180/105 mmHg, and there was some tenderness in the left loin associated with a mild degree of spasm in the left paravertebral muscles at the thoracolumbar junction. Trunk mobility was restricted on side-bending to the right, and was associated with pain in the left thoracolumbar area. Otherwise, the physical examination was quite normal.

Questions for discussion

- Do the findings on physical examination help you in your assessment of Mrs Kendall's problem?
- What causes can you think of for moderate hypertension that might be relevant to Mrs Kendall?
- Which investigations do you think might be useful at this stage to elucidate the problem?
- What would you tell Mrs Kendall?
- What therapy would you give Mrs Kendall at this stage?

A blood test was ordered for Mrs Kendall, and revealed the following results:

Full blood count	Normal
Erythrocyte sedimentation rate	20 mm in first hour
Plasma sodium	139 mmol l^{-1}
Plasma potassium	4.5 mmol l^{-1}
Plasma chloride	100 mmol l^{-1}
Plasma bicarbonate	26 mmol l^{-1}
Plasma urea	7.0 mmol l^{-1}
Serum calcium	2.9 mmol l^{-1}
Serum phosphate	0.8 mmol l^{-1}
Serum albumin	42 g l^{-1}

   A plain X-ray of the lumbar spine was reported as showing calcification in the abdomen, most likely to be in the kidneys. There was no obvious bony pathology in the lumbar spine.

Questions for discussion

- Which of the blood test results are abnormal?

- Do the results of these investigations help you with your diagnosis of Mrs Kendall's problem?

- How do you think the high serum calcium and the kidney calcification are related?

- How might Mrs Kendall's hypertension be related to the X-ray findings?

- Are there any other investigations that you would like to order for Mrs Kendall?

In order to understand Mrs Kendall's problem more fully, it is necessary for you to study the metabolism of calcium and its relationship with the kidney (see also Ch. 14 for more activities on calcium and bone metabolism).

Activity 13.11

▶ You will need a measuring jug which holds approximately 1 litre for this activity. (The activity will take several days to complete, so you will need to be patient and conscientious.) Measure the intake of fluid and the volume of urine that you produce in a 24-hour period.

▶ Repeat this a few times to see how variable the result is.

▶ Repeat the measurement after drinking an extra 2 or 3 litres of (non-alcoholic) fluid during the day.

▶ If you drink alcohol, you might like to see if this makes any difference. Try drinking a very moderate amount of beer (say 1 or 2 pints) and measuring the urine output over the next 24 hours. Compare this with drinking the same number of units of alcohol, but in whisky or other spirits, so that the volume of fluid is much smaller (a pint of beer is about 2 units of alcohol, while a 25 ml measure of whisky is about 1 unit).

▶ If you have access to a very accurate pair of scales, you might also like to weigh yourself at intervals after drinking.

▶ Now drink a quantity of about 1–2 litres of water, and measure the urine output each hour for a few hours afterwards. (You don't need to pass urine on the hour, just note down the output over the period of 1 hour.)

▶ You could repeat this with the alcohol if you wish. If you have access to laboratory testing facilities, you could even test the urine for specific gravity or concentration of, for example, sodium and potassium.

Questions for discussion

- What happens to the urine output when you drink extra fluid?
- Does alcohol have any measurable effect on urine output?

Activity 13.12

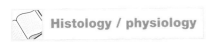 Histology / physiology

▶ Study the structure and function of the kidney. Note that the functional unit is called a nephron, and note that it consists essentially of:
    — A glomerulus, which filters the blood
    — A tubule, in which the filtrate is modified to become urine.
▶ Note the arrangement of the arterial supply to the glomerulus and to the tubules, with the afferent and efferent arterioles supplying the glomerulus and the vasa recta dipping down into the kidney medulla to supply the loop of Henle.
▶ Note the proximal tubule, the arrangement of the descending and ascending limb of the loop of Henle, the distal tubule and the collecting duct on its way to the renal pelvis.
▶ Study the structure of the cells in each of these regions of the nephron.
▶ Note that the basic mechanism by which the kidney eliminates excess waste products is as follows:
    — Approximately 20% of the blood flowing through the glomerulus is filtered into the tubular system
    — The tubular system reabsorbs the substances which are required, while the waste products stay in the tubules to be excreted as urine
    — A small amount of secretion of waste products occurs into the tubular fluid via the cells lining the tubules.

Questions for discussion

- What do you think is the significance of the fact that the pressure in glomerular blood vessels is high while pressure in tubular blood vessels is low?

- What is meant by the term 'glomerular filtration rate' (GFR)?
- What is the normal composition of glomerular filtrate compared with blood plasma?
- How does the glomerular membrane allow large quantities of fluid and small molecules to enter the tubular fluid, while restricting the passage of large molecules such as proteins?
- How do you think that the glomerular filtration rate would be affected by constriction of
  - the afferent arteriole
  - the efferent arteriole?

Activity 13.13

▶ Study the dynamics of tubular reabsorption of substances that have been filtered at the glomeruli.

More than 99% of the water in the filtrate is reabsorbed, so that the urine flow rate is about 1 ml per minute while the GFR is about 120 ml per minute. Some molecules, such as glucose and amino acids, are completely reabsorbed, so that their urine concentration is zero. Tubular reabsorption may involve:

— Active transport, which involves the expenditure of energy

— Passive transport, in which no energy is expended.

The active transport mainly involves the transport of sodium ions from the tubular cell into the kidney interstitium. This leads to diffusion of sodium ions from the tubular lumen. This process also energises other 'carrier' mechanisms that transport molecules such as glucose and amino acids. Note particularly for the purposes of this case that calcium and magnesium are actively reabsorbed in the tubules.

Questions for discussion

- What do you understand by the term 'tubular load' of a substance?
- What do you understand by the term 'tubular transport maximum' of an actively reabsorbed or secreted substance?
- What percentage of the calcium that enters the glomerular filtrate remains in the distal tubules?

In the next activity you are going to study the regulation of the blood concentration of calcium (see also Ch. 14 for further activities on calcium and bone).

Activity 13.14

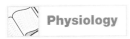 **Physiology**

▶ Study the absorption and excretion of calcium in the body. Note that calcium is relatively poorly absorbed from the gut because many calcium compounds are insoluble. Note the effect of vitamin D as it increases the formation of a calcium-binding protein in the epithelial cells of the intestines. This increases the active transport of calcium into the intestinal cells, and the calcium can then be transported across the basolateral membrane of the cells by facilitated diffusion. Note particularly the chemical reactions that are involved in the formation of the active form of vitamin D, and note that both the liver and the kidney must be functioning for the reactions to occur satisfactorily.

▶ Now study the calcium in the plasma and the interstitial fluid. The concentration of calcium in the plasma is approximately 2.4 mmol l^{-1}, and the level is quite closely regulated by a negative feedback mechanism.

To illustrate the action of a negative feedback mechanism, think of what happens when you drive a car at a constant speed, say 50 km per hour. You look at the speedometer to check that you are travelling at the correct speed. If you are travelling too fast, the speedometer will tell you so and you will ease your foot off the accelerator until the speedometer reads 50. Conversely, if you are travelling too slowly the speedometer will read below 50 and you will increase your pressure on the accelerator until the speed is once more correct. The amount of variation above and below the correct level will depend on many factors, not least of which is how often you look at the speedometer and how much you are prepared to let the speed deviate from 50.

 If you analyse what is going on in this example, you will find that there are several components:

— There is a speed at which you desire to travel

— There is a device (the speedometer) for detecting the actual speed of the car

— You compare the actual speed of the car with the desired speed

— If you are travelling at the desired speed, you change nothing

— If you are travelling at a different speed from that desired, you put into effect a change in pressure on the accelerator until the speed matches the desired level

— You continue to compare the actual speed with the desired speed and repeat the previous three steps.

Any negative feedback mechanism has the same basic principle. The components are:

— A controlled variable (car speed)

— A detector (speedometer) for detecting the actual level of the controlled variable

— A comparator (you) for comparing the actual level of the controlled variable with the desired level

— An error signal, which results when the actual level is different from the desired level

— An effector (accelerator pedal) for correcting any discrepancy between actual and desired levels.

The same concepts can be applied to the regulation of the plasma calcium level, and will be discussed a little later in this case study. First, note that calcium is present in different forms in the plasma:

— Bound to plasma proteins (approx 40%)

— Combined with other ions (approx 10%)

— Ionised (approx 50%).

Questions for discussion

■ What are the major sources of calcium in the diet?

■ How much calcium is provided per day by an average western diet?

■ How much calcium is absorbed per day by an average adult?

■ Which factors affect the amount of calcium absorbed via the intestines?

■ What are the major functions of calcium in the various body systems?

■ Which form of calcium is important for these functions?

■ Vitamin D_3 has been termed a hormone. Give reasons why you would agree or disagree with this.

Activity 13.15

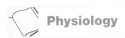 Physiology

▶ Now you need to study the negative feedback mechanism for control of the blood calcium level. Study the structure and functions of the parathyroid glands. Note that there are usually four parathyroid glands, situated just behind the thyroid gland. Study the position, size and blood supply of the glands. Note:

— The histological structure of the glands, with an abundance of chief cells and a minority of oxyphil cells in the adult

— The chemistry of parathyroid hormone (PTH); it is a polypeptide with 84 amino acids.

The effect of a rise in the blood level of PTH is a rise in the blood calcium level and a decrease in the phosphate level. The effect on calcium is due mainly to:

— Release of calcium (and phosphate) from bone

— Decrease in calcium excretion by the kidney.

   The effect on phosphate is due mainly to increased renal excretion, which predominates over the release from bone tending to increase plasma phosphate levels. (The effect of PTH on bone is discussed further in Ch. 14.) PTH increases tubular reabsorption of calcium by increasing the active transport mechanisms in the renal tubules.

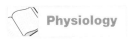 Physiology

▶ Now study how PTH itself is controlled.

The main factor in this control is the level of calcium in the blood, in that even a slight rise in blood calcium will cause a fall in PTH secretion. Conversely, anything that causes a decrease in plasma calcium levels will cause the parathyroid glands to increase their production of PTH. The effect is even more pronounced if the calcium levels have been low for a period of weeks, because the glands can hypertrophy and so become more sensitive to small changes in the plasma calcium level.

Question for discussion

■ What is the effect of PTH on intestinal absorption of calcium and phosphate?

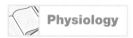
Physiology

▶ To complicate the issue a little, it is necessary for you to study the effects of a hormone called calcitonin, which is produced in the thyroid gland. Study the structure and actions of calcitonin. Note that it is produced in the C cells of the thyroid gland, and is a polypeptide with 32 amino acids. Its main effect is to reduce plasma calcium by:

— Increasing deposition of calcium in bone

— Decreasing resorption of bone by the osteoclasts.

In general, the effects of calcitonin are opposite to those of PTH, although it has a less powerful and more rapid action. In children, when bone turnover is much higher than in the adult, the importance of calcitonin is increased. Its secretion is also controlled by the plasma calcium level, but in the opposite direction to that of PTH.

Question for discussion

■ What effect does removal of the thyroid gland have on plasma calcium concentration?

Activity 13.16

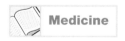
Medicine

▶ Now you need to study the causes and clinical features of hypercalcaemia. First look at the causes of hypercalcaemia (see also Ch. 10 for further discussion of hypercalcaemia). Note that there are many causes, including:

— Hyperparathyroidism

— Malignancy, e.g. myeloma, lymphoma, carcinoma, leukaemia

— Sarcoidosis

— Milk–alkali syndrome.

Questions for discussion

■ Why might a high calcium level be an artefact?

■ Which of the conditions causing hypercalcaemia are associated with an increased level of the active form of vitamin D?

■ Why might the PTH levels be low in someone with a tumour which is destroying bone?

Note that some tumours can secrete a PTH-like peptide (so-called 'ectopic hormone' production) which elevates plasma calcium.

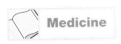 **Medicine**

▶ Study the clinical features of hypercalcaemia. Note that mild hypercalcaemia may give rise to no symptoms at all, but marked hypercalcaemia is a medical emergency. The main symptoms of hypercalcaemia include:

— Thirst, polyuria, polydipsia

— Constipation, abdominal discomfort, anorexia, nausea, vomiting

— Depression, lethargy, psychosis.

Note that ectopic calcification is common with any cause of hypercalcaemia. The kidneys are particularly subject to calcification in the form of stones.

Questions for discussion

■ What other sites are liable to ectopic calcification?

■ What is the effect of hypercalcaemia on the cardiovascular system?

■ Which investigations might differentiate the causes of hypercalcaemia from one another?

Activity 13.17

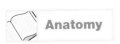 **Anatomy**

▶ If you are not familiar with the structures in the abdomen, you should revise the basic anatomy before you study the film in your textbook.

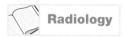 **Radiology**

▶ Look at an abdominal X-ray. It is called a 'plain' abdominal X-ray because no extra material has been added to outline the various structures. As with any radiograph, it is necessary to have a methodical sequence when you study the plain abdominal X-ray. It is important to note that you see structures outlined only when there is a difference in radiodensity at the margins of the structure.

▶ Compare the abdominal film with a chest X-ray and note that the outline of the heart is quite clear, because the fluid in the heart has a different density from the air in the lungs. In the plain abdominal film, the layer of fat around the kidneys, for example, may provide a relatively radiolucent layer which can outline the shape of the kidneys. If there is inflammation around the kidneys, this difference in density disappears and the kidneys are no longer seen so easily.

As long as your method of studying the X-ray includes all the structures, it may not matter in which order you do it, but a fairly logical method is as follows:

— The spine. Look at the layers of vertebral body (like a box), pedicles (circles outlined in white), spinous process (teardrop shape) and articular processes ('wings' of bone). Note the different structures in turn and note also whether there is symmetry of the structures

— The ribs. You will see the lower ribs fairly clearly

— The pelvis and femoral head and neck. You should note that there are shadows from air in the intestines. It may sometimes be difficult to distinguish these from pathological erosions of bone

— The organs. The size of the liver on a plain radiograph is not a good indication of its size, whereas that of the spleen is a better guide. Note the stomach, with its air bubble. The gallbladder may be visible on the plain film. The kidney outline can often be traced fairly well, but it is often obscured by intestinal gas shadows. The pancreas is not well visualised unless there is calcification in it. Note the loops of small and large intestine, with the colon being better outlined because of its air content. The bladder may be visible as a rounded shadow in the pelvis

— The soft tissues. Note the 'flank stripe' where the X-ray beam catches the fatty layer next to the abdominal wall tangentially. This may be obscured when there is local inflammation. Look for the psoas shadow extending down from the kidney area. Look for calcifications, which could be stones, calcified thrombi, phleboliths or calcified lymph nodes.

Questions for discussion

- How does lying a patient prone for an abdominal X-ray affect the appearance of the stomach bubble?
- In terms of X-ray densities, why is it easy to see the hip joint?

Activity 13.18

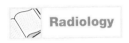 **Radiology**

▶ Now look at an intravenous urogram (IVU).

Clearly, the main difference between this X-ray film and the plain abdominal film is that the kidneys are opaque and well defined. To achieve this, an injection of a radio-opaque substance is injected intravenously. This substance is excreted in the glomerular filtrate and not reabsorbed, so its concentration in the tubular fluid rises and the radiodensity of the kidneys increases above that of the surroundings. In a normally functioning kidney, the shadow of the renal parenchyma whitens significantly after only about a minute; after this, the dye proceeds down the calyces, pelves and ureters, and most of the dye is in the bladder by around 30 minutes.

If there is obstruction to the flow of urine, for example by a stone in the ureter, the appearance of the dye is delayed and the density of the affected kidney is reduced.

Questions for discussion

- Why do you not see the entire length of the ureters in a single film?
- What other imaging techniques might be useful for demonstrating kidney problems?

Investigation

The IVU in Mrs Kendall was reported as showing stones in the left kidney. The parathyroid hormone level in the blood was $3.0\ \mu g\ ml^{-1}$ (normal range < 0.8). A diagnosis of primary hyperparathyroidism was therefore made.

Questions for discussion

- What effect does immobility have on the hypercalcaemia of hyperparathyroidism?
- What is the characteristic bone disease associated with hyperparathyroidism?
- How would you manage Mrs Kendall?

Discussion

Low back pain is a symptom with a multitude of causes. As with most symptoms which present to a manual therapist, the first question to ask is whether the pain is arising from a mechanical problem in the painful area, or whether the pain is referred from a distant structure (or indeed whether both possibilities exist at the same time).

Mrs Kendall has features that should make you think of a non-mechanical reason for her pain. The most obvious feature is the passing of gravel in the urine, which is associated with the formation of stones in the urinary tract. Pain arising in the kidney generally is felt in the loin, and ureteric pain extends from the loin to the groin. When you realise that Mrs Kendall may be forming kidney stones, the next question is why. Some of the other symptoms that Mrs Kendall has noticed may then be considered as more relevant to the problem as a whole.

It has been estimated that approximately 1% of the population of the UK will have symptomatic urinary stones at some stage in their life. Most stones in the urinary tract contain calcium, but a small minority contain uric acid (which is associated with gout) or cystine. These substances are not very soluble, and can precipitate out in the urine under the conditions occurring there. Most people with calcium stones have a normal blood calcium level, but many will have an increase in urinary calcium excretion. Mrs Kendall also has hypercalcaemia, and so underlying causes such as hyperparathyroidism, sarcoidosis, vitamin D intoxication, malignant disease or hyperthyroidism must be considered.

Hypercalcaemia may be asymptomatic if it is mild. More severe degrees of hypercalcaemia may cause symptoms in the renal, gastrointestinal and neurological systems. These may be quite vague, and be ascribed to 'general wear and tear' or the ageing process. On reviewing Mrs Kendall's history, it is clear that many of her previous symptoms could have been attributed to hypercalcaemia.

Investigation of a patient with hypercalcaemia aims to elucidate the various causes. A full blood count may reveal anaemia, and a markedly raised ESR or plasma viscosity may suggest myeloma or cancer. A chest X-ray may suggest a primary or secondary lung cancer or sarcoidosis. Plasma levels of parathyroid hormone are raised in primary hyperparathyroidism, and this was the case with Mrs Kendall. There are more complicated diagnostic techniques to localise a parathyroid tumour which you may care to look up in your textbooks.

The most dramatic presentation of a stone in the urinary tract is with the intense pain of renal or ureteric colic, which results from the complete obstruction of urinary flow. However, many patients report only mild discomfort in the loin area, perhaps associated with the passing of gravel in the urine. Mild haematuria is a frequent accompaniment to this, and should always prompt a thorough investigation for more serious causes.

Mrs Kendall presented with left loin discomfort, and a history of passing gravel. Blood analysis revealed hypercalcaemia, and abdominal X-ray and IVU revealed renal stones. The plasma PTH was raised. A diagnosis of primary hyperparathyroidism was thus made. She had a computerised tomogram to localise the tumour and subsequently underwent parathyroid surgery, with a successful result.

FURTHER READING

Chan A K, Duh Q Y, Katz M H, Siperstein A E, Clark O H 1995 Clinical manifestations of primary hyperparathyroidism before and after parathyroidectomy. A case-control study. Annals of Surgery 222: 402–412

Mrs Eileen Thomas

After studying this case with its associated activities and questions, you should have a reasonable knowledge of the following areas:

1. Surface anatomy of structures in the pelvic area
2. Gross anatomy of the hip bone
3. Gross anatomy of the sacrum
4. Anatomy of the bony pelvis as a whole
5. Structure of the sacroiliac joint
6. Attachments and functions of the ligaments of the pelvis
7. Attachments, actions, blood and nerve supply of the muscles attached to the bony pelvis
8. Blood vessels of the pelvis
9. Lymphatic drainage of the pelvic structures
10. Gross anatomy of the sacral plexus of nerves
11. Anatomy of the nerves supplying the pelvic structures
12. Biomechanics of sacroiliac joint movements
13. Performing standing and seated flexion tests
14. Assessing symmetry and mobility of the bony pelvis
15. Causes of pain in the sacroiliac region
16. Histology of bone
17. Physiology of bone formation and resorption
18. Effects of hormones on bone turnover
19. Pathology of osteoporosis
20. Causes and clinical features of osteoporosis
21. Principles of prevention of osteoporosis
22. Management of a patient with established osteoporosis.

Background

The husband of Mrs Eileen Thomas, a 69-year-old housewife, telephoned your surgery one Friday morning in a rather distressed state. Mrs Thomas had turned over in bed the previous night and had experienced a sudden shooting pain across her low back and into the top of her right buttock. She found it extremely difficult to move at all, and would appreciate a home visit. Mrs Thomas was an old patient of yours, and before you drove to her house you looked at her notes and reminded yourself of her history. Since you had just had a very busy day, and were due to go to a meeting later that evening, you decided just to review the outline of her history, and leave the details until you talked to her at her home.

You noted that she had suffered from thoracic pain for some time in the past 10 years, and that osteoporosis had been diagnosed some 5 years previously. She had been taking hormone replacement therapy since the diagnosis, as well as calcium and vitamin D supplements, and simple analgesia to be taken as required.

Questions for discussion

- What are your thoughts on Mrs Thomas's problem as you drive to her house?
- What questions would you like to ask her when you get to see her?

When you arrived at Mrs Thomas's home, you were met by her husband who was very relieved indeed to see you. As you went up the stairs to her bedroom, he told you that she had been unable to get out of bed all day, and had consumed a large quantity of her painkillers.

Mrs Thomas herself told you that the pain was a sharp, shooting pain located mainly across the lumbosacral region, worse on the right side and extending into the right buttock. It was quite different from the pains that she had experienced in the past from her osteoporosis, which was a dull aching sensation, and she found it difficult to get out of bed without a moderately severe muscle spasm in her low back. There was no radiation of pain further down the leg, and there were no pins and needles and no loss of sensation in the leg. It was difficult for her to tell whether or not there was any loss of muscle power because every time she tried to move, the spasms made it difficult for her to get anywhere.

From her case records, you noted that she had not visited you for about 3 years, and she confirmed that she had been quite well during that period, only needing to take her painkillers on very infrequent occasions and being able to take long walks across the moor without much discomfort. Her appetite was good and her weight steady, she did not have any cough, wheeze or shortness of breath, and there was no pain in the chest or abdomen. Bowel motions and passing urine did not give her any trouble, although she had found it difficult to move her bowels that day because of the pain. Further general enquiry did not reveal any abnormal symptoms.

Questions for discussion

- How does Mrs Thomas's osteoporosis influence the way you think about her present problem?
- On which aspects of the physical examination would you like to concentrate?

Activity 14.1

▶ You will need your partner undressed to his underpants for this activity. Identify the following structures on your partner's lower trunk (if the structure is bilateral, compare right and left sides):

— Iliac crest

— Anterior superior iliac spine (ASIS)

— Inguinal ligament

— Femoral artery pulsation

— Pubic tubercle

— Body of pubis

— Symphysis pubis

— Spines of 4th and 5th lumbar vertebrae

— Posterior superior iliac spine (PSIS)

— Spines of sacrum

— Coccyx

— Ischial tuberosity

— Inferior lateral angle of the sacrum (ILA)

— Gluteal fold.

Question for discussion

■ What differences can you think of between a male and a female pelvis?

Activity 14.2

▶ Have your partner, still undressed, stand facing away from you. Place your right thumb on the inferior aspect of his right PSIS. Repeat with your left thumb on his left PSIS. Ask your partner to slowly bend forwards from the waist, with his legs straight, as if to touch his toes. As your partner bends forwards, note the movement of the PSIS, comparing each side. Note whether the PSIS on the right side is initially at the same horizontal level as that on the left. This test is known as a 'standing flexion test'.

Questions for discussion

■ How would you interpret the finding that the right PSIS was initially higher than the left?

■ How would you interpret the finding that the right PSIS moved further than the left on forward bending?

▶ Have your partner seated with his back to you on a stool. The stool should be low enough to allow his feet to touch the floor, with his feet and knees about 50 cm apart. Ask your partner to lace his fingers behind his neck and put his elbows forward. You should kneel behind him, with your thumbs on each PSIS in a similar fashion to the standing position, and ask him to bend forwards from the waist as far as he can comfortably go. The elbows should be able to move down between the knees. Observe the movement of each PSIS and compare the two sides as before. This is known as the 'seated flexion test'.

Question for discussion

■ How would you interpret the finding that the right PSIS moved further than the left on forward bending in the seated flexion test?

Activity 14.3

▶ Have your partner lie supine on an examination couch. Palpate the ASIS on each side simultaneously, placing the pads of your thumbs under the bony protuberance. Assess whether one ASIS is superior/inferior or anterior/posterior relative to the other.

▶ Bring the pads of your index fingers along the inguinal ligament to the superior aspect of your partner's pubic tubercles. Note the relative position of your fingers and assess whether one is superior.

▶ Ask your partner to flex his knees so that both feet are flat on the couch. He should then raise his buttocks and lower them. You then extend his legs and note the relative position of the medial malleoli by placing your thumbs under the distal prominence. You then put your partner's right leg through a series of manoeuvres:
 — Flex the hip and knee
 — Externally rotate and abduct the hip
 — Extend the leg.

▶ Compare again the relative position of the medial malleoli.

▶ Repeat the series of manoeuvres, with the second movement being internal rotation and adduction rather than external rotation and abduction.

▶ Again, compare the position of the medial malleoli.

Questions for discussion

■ What happens to the relative position of the medial malleoli when you perform the manoeuvres on your partner's leg?

■ Try to explain the mechanism of any changes that you observe.

▶ Ask your partner to turn over and lie prone on the couch. Palpate the PSIS on each side by placing your thumbs on the inferior ledge, and assess whether one PSIS is superior/inferior or anterior/posterior relative to the other. Slide your thumbs medially and into the sacral sulci, assessing the relative depth on each side. Palpate the inferior lateral angles of the sacrum and again assess whether one is superior/inferior or anterior/posterior relative to the other.

▶ Place the heel of your right hand on your partner's lower lumbar spine and the heel of your left hand on top of your right hand. Exert gentle downward pressure on the spine and note the resistance to your pressure.

The assessment of the relative positions of the various structures mentioned in Activities 14.2 and 14.3 is not easy, and requires a lot of practice under the supervision of an experienced teacher. However, the only way to become competent in this as in any other activity, is to practise many times, using different people in order to develop a feel for the range of 'normality'.

▶ Try to develop your skill in assessing whether a structure on one side is higher than its fellow on the other side by putting two nails about 50 cm apart and nearly at the same height above the ground. Estimate which is higher, and check your estimation using a spirit level.

▶ Or attach a small spirit level to a piece of stiff wire which can be placed on both iliac crests to check your assessment of the relative height of these structures in the living body.

Activity 14.4

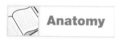 **Anatomy**

▶ Now it is time to take a more detailed look at the structure and function of the pelvis. Study a picture of the pelvis. Note its resemblance to a basin (pelvis is the Latin for basin). Note the hip bone, consisting of the ilium, ischium and pubis, noting particularly the following:

— Acetabulum on the lateral surface

— Obturator foramen

— Iliac crest

— Anterior superior iliac spine

— Posterior superior iliac spine

— Auricular surface of the ilium

— Pubic crest

— Pubic tubercle

— Pubic symphysis
— Superior and inferior rami of the pubis
— Ischial tuberosity
— Ischial spine.

▶ Now study the sacrum, noting in particular the following features:

— Apex
— Base, which is similar to a typical lumbar vertebra
— Sacral promontory
— Median sacral crest
— Sacral cornua
— Inferior lateral angles
— Auricular surface, for articulation with the ilium.

▶ Look at the pelvis as a whole, with hip bone and sacrum articulated. Note:

— The inclination of the pelvis in the living person when in the upright position
— The superior pelvic aperture (pelvic inlet) and inferior pelvic aperture (pelvic outlet); note that each aperture has an anteroposterior and a transverse diameter, and that the inlet also has an oblique diameter.

Questions for discussion

■ What is the importance of measuring the various pelvic diameters in the female?

■ How do the differences between the male and female pelvis relate to child bearing?

Activity 14.5

▶ While you are studying the bony pelvis, it is useful to think about its function in supporting the abdomen and providing a link between the legs and the trunk.

The weight of the upper body is transmitted via the 5th lumbar vertebra, along the sacrum and ilia towards the acetabula. The force from the reaction of the ground travels up the femora and then divides into a force meeting the downward force from the trunk and another travelling across the pubic rami to be counterbalanced by a similar force from the other side. There is therefore a complete ring of force lines around the pelvic brim. If you look at an X-ray of the pelvic bones, you will note that the bony trabeculae form a system of lines which correspond to the lines of force.

▶ Study the articular surfaces of the ilium and sacrum which comprise the sacroiliac joint.

The iliac surface, lying on the medial surface of the ilium, near the iliopectineal line, is shaped somewhat like a boomerang, with its concavity facing posteriorly. The articular surface is quite irregular, but you might imagine it to be like a railway embankment curved in an arc of a circle, with the centre of the circle being near the iliac tuberosity. The iliac surface of the sacroiliac joint is covered in hyaline cartilage. There is a correspondingly shaped sacral surface, with its valley-like shape in a similar curve to that on the ilium. It is covered in fibrocartilage. The centre of the sacral curve lies near to the transverse process element of the 2nd sacral vertebra. Note, however, that this comparison with a circle is very approximate and the 'embankment–valley' comparison only holds at certain portions of the surfaces.

A further complexity is that the sacrum with its articular surface varies widely between individuals. Occasionally, the left and right sacroiliac joints are not the same shape in the same person!

Questions for discussion

- How does the shape of the sacrum vary with the degree of lordosis of the lumbar vertebral column?
- Can you think of any functional significance that such variation might have?
- Why is the strain on the lumbosacral joint greater if a person has an increased lumbar lordosis?

▶ Have your partner stand with his back to you and resting his weight evenly on both legs. If you have two sets of bathroom scales, you can check whether his weight is symmetrically distributed by having him put each foot on a set of scales and noting the readings – they should be equal.

▶ Now get a block of wood just larger than your partner's foot and about 3 cm thick and place it under your partner's right foot. Ask him if this arrangement feels uncomfortable, and repeat the measurements on the scales.

▶ Note whether your partner's spine has curved to compensate for the tilting of the pelvis.

▶ Try repeating this exercise with blocks of wood of various thicknesses.

Questions for discussion

■ What do you think would happen to the distribution of force in the pelvic ring in a person who
  – had one leg longer than the other
  – was carrying a baby on her hip?

Activity 14.6

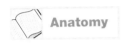 Anatomy

▶ Study the ligaments of the pelvis. Note the attachments of the following ligaments:
  — Iliolumbar
  — Ventral sacroiliac
  — Interosseous sacroiliac
  — Dorsal sacroiliac
  — Sacrotuberous
  — Sacrospinous
  — Superior pubic
  — Arcuate pubic.

▶ Observe the direction of the fibres of the ligaments, and how they become taut with various movements. Note how the sacroiliac ligaments are wrapped around the joint, and try to work out which movements they will allow.

▶ Look at a whole spine, and imagine the forces that occur on the lumbosacral joint during standing.

▶ Note how the sacrotuberous and sacrospinous ligaments oppose the forward movement of the sacral base in the upright posture.

▶ Now study the movements at the sacroiliac joint.

It has to be said at the outset that this is a most controversial issue, and there are many authorities who do not believe that movement occurs at the adult sacroiliac joint except during labour. In any case, the range of movement is extremely small, is slightly greater in the pregnant female, and varies between individuals and even in the same individual under different conditions. It is therefore very difficult to obtain consistent results when studying the movements of this joint, and various therapists have their own pet theories about what they are doing when they treat problems arising in the area.

▶ Firstly, study the movement known as 'nutation'. In this, the sacral promontory moves downwards and forwards while the apex of the sacrum (together with the coccyx) moves backwards. The axis of rotation is through the interosseous sacroiliac ligament.

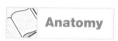 **Anatomy**

▶ If you have access to a bony or plastic pelvis, try to imitate this movement. If you do not, look at a picture in your textbook and imagine the effect of the movement.

In 'nutation' the anteroposterior diameter of the pelvic inlet is reduced, while that of the outlet is increased. Also, because of the triangular cross-sectional shape of the sacrum, the iliac bones tend to come closer together and the ischial tuberosities move further apart.

The movement of 'counter-nutation' is the opposite of nutation, with the sacral promontory moving upwards and backwards, and the apex and coccyx moving forwards. At the same time, the iliac bones move apart and the ischial tuberosities move together.

Questions for discussion

■ Which ligaments limit the movements of nutation and counter-nutation?

■ Do you know of any other possible axes of rotation of the sacroiliac joint?

■ Is there a difference between sacral motion on the ilium and ilial motion on the sacrum?

■ What happens to the pelvic ligaments during pregnancy and labour?

■ Which movements occur at the sacroiliac joint during walking?

■ Compare the structure and function of the pectoral girdle with the pelvic girdle.

▶ Look at the structure of the pubic symphysis. It is a secondary cartilaginous joint, with the ends of the two opposing pubic bones being lined by hyaline cartilage and joined by fibrocartilage. The articular surface is oval. Note the strength of the ligaments supporting the joint.

Question for discussion

■ Which muscles are attached to the pubic symphysis?

The movements that are allowed at this joint are:

— Sliding

— Separation.

In practice, there is very little movement at this joint, but it is subject to considerable strain during standing and walking. Again, the ligaments become lax during pregnancy and labour, and allow for separation of the pubic bones and thus enlargement of the pelvic cavity.

▶ Finally in this activity, look at the sacrococcygeal joint. This is also a secondary cartilaginous joint, and the movements available are passive flexion and extension. During nutation, the coccyx helps to enlarge the pelvic outlet as it amplifies the movement of the sacrum.

Activity 14.7

▶ The muscles of the pelvic region do not directly move the sacroiliac joint or the pubis; they are used for moving the trunk or the legs. Revise the attachments, actions, nerve supply and blood supply of the muscles attached to the pelvis.

There are many of these muscles, and so it is probably useful to think of them in groups.

Anterolateral muscles of the abdomen

— Internal oblique

— External oblique

— Rectus abdominis

— Transversus abdominis

— Pyramidalis.

The actions of this group of muscles include opposing the action of gravity on the abdominal viscera and assisting in fixing the abdomen during respiration. They increase intra-abdominal pressure and so aid in expelling faeces from the rectum and the fetus during childbirth. They help to bend the trunk forwards and flex the lumbar spine if the pelvis is fixed; if the upper trunk is fixed, they help to rotate the pelvis upwards. Muscles acting unilaterally help to side-bend the trunk to that side. These muscles also help to form the curve of the waist.

Questions for discussion

■ Which muscles do you use when you rotate the trunk?

■ How do these muscles help to protect the lumbosacral disc when lifting a heavy weight?

Posterior muscles of the abdomen

— Psoas major

— Psoas minor

— Iliacus

— Quadratus lumborum.

Note the actions of the psoas major and iliacus in flexing the thigh on the pelvis and in bending the trunk forwards in a similar way to the anterolateral group. Note particularly the role of the psoas muscle in accentuating the lumbar lordosis. These muscles do not directly contribute to the increase in abdominal pressure. Note the action of quadratus lumborum in fixing the 12th rib and steadying the diaphragm during respiration. One quadratus lumborum muscle acting unilaterally side-bends the trunk to the side of the active muscle, while both acting together tend to extend the lumbar spine.

Posterior trunk muscles

— Erector spinae

— Multifidus.

Note the action of these muscles as trunk extensors, but also in increasing the lumbar lordosis.

Muscles of the pelvis and perineum

— Levator ani
— Coccygeus
— Bulbospongiosus
— Ischiocavernosus.

These muscles are important in the support of the pelvic floor and the function of the pelvic viscera. Note the actions of the individual muscles in defaecation, micturition, childbirth and sexual activity.

Anterior femoral muscles

— Tensor fasciae latae
— Sartorius
— Rectus femoris.

Note the actions of these muscles in steadying the pelvis on the femur during standing, and in flexing the thigh on the pelvis during walking.

Medial femoral muscles

— Gracilis
— Pectineus
— Adductor longus
— Adductor brevis
— Adductor magnus.

Note the actions of these muscles as adductors of the thigh as well as flexors of the thigh on the pelvis. The adductors also produce lateral rotation of the femur, while the gracilis produces medial rotation.

Muscles of the gluteal region

— Gluteus maximus
— Gluteus medius
— Gluteus minimus
— Piriformis
— Obturator internus
— Obturator externus

— Gemellus superior

— Gemellus inferior

— Quadratus femoris.

Note the actions of the gluteus muscles in extending and abducting the thigh; they are particularly important in walking. The other muscles are mainly external rotators of the femur.

Question for discussion

- If a patient had a paralysis of the right gluteus medius, what would happen if you asked him to stand on his right leg?

Posterior femoral muscles

— Biceps femoris

— Semitendinosus

— Semimembranosus.

Note the action of these muscles supporting the pelvis on the head of the femur. The biceps femoris can act as a lateral rotator of the leg, whereas the other two muscles in this group act as medial rotators.

Questions for discussion

- Which muscles are used when you rise from a stooping position?
- Which muscles are used when you stand upright with the weight evenly distributed over both feet?
- How do the muscles react when you stand with your weight predominantly on one foot? Is there any difference in the muscular action if you lift one foot completely off the ground?

You will have gathered from the number of muscles that act on the pelvis and the diversity of their actions, that the pelvis is a very important structure in the maintenance of the erect posture. It is an important region for you to study carefully.

Activity 14.8

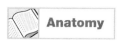 **Anatomy**

▶ Study the blood supply of the pelvis. The main artery in this region is the internal iliac artery, a branch of the common iliac artery (see also Ch. 3). Note that this artery arises in front of the sacroiliac joint, and note its close relationship with the lumbosacral nerve trunk as well as the sacroiliac joint, with the ureter and, in the female, with the ovary and Fallopian tube.

▶ Follow the artery to the upper edge of the greater sciatic foramen, where it divides into an anterior and a posterior trunk.

▶ Follow the anterior trunk towards the ischial spine, and the posterior trunk which curves backwards towards the greater sciatic foramen.

▶ Note its branches to the pelvic structures, and in particular note the course and supply of the following:

— Obturator artery

— Inferior gluteal artery

— Lateral sacral arteries

— Superior gluteal artery.

▶ Note that the external iliac artery gives off branches to some of the muscles of the lower abdomen and a few pelvic structures, but that its main claim to fame is that it continues as the femoral artery (see also Ch. 3).

▶ Look at the internal and external iliac veins, and their relation to the corresponding arteries. In the main, the tributaries of the internal iliac vein correspond with the branches of the artery. Note particularly the plexuses of veins around the rectum, prostate, vagina, uterus and bladder.

Questions for discussion

■ What happens if the veins of the rectal plexus become dilated and varicose?

■ Why may portal hypertension cause haemorrhoids?

▶ Study the lymphatic drainage of the pelvis. It is important to have a knowledge of this in order to be able to predict the spread of cancer in this region. Note particularly the drainage of the rectum and anus, the lower urinary tract, the reproductive organs and the lower abdominal wall.

Question for discussion

■ Which cancers of pelvic organs spread to bone?

Activity 14.9

▶ Now it is time for you to pluck up courage and study the nerves in the pelvic region. Actually, it is not too difficult. Ask your partner to strip to his underpants.

▶ Ask him to perform the following movements while lying supine:
— Hip flexion ('lift your leg')
— Hip adduction ('move your legs apart')
— Hip abduction ('press your legs together')
— Hip external rotation ('turn your feet outwards')
— Hip internal rotation ('turn your feet inwards')
— Trunk flexion ('lift your shoulders off the couch').

▶ Ask your partner to turn over into the prone position, and ask him to perform hip extension by lifting his leg off the couch with the knee kept extended.

▶ Test the sensation of the skin around the lower abdomen and lower part of the posterior aspect of the trunk (see also Chs 6 and 7). Test the skin with a piece of cotton wool and the point of a sterile pin and mark out the dermatomes from T10–L2 and from S2–S4.

Questions for discussion

■ Which nerve root levels supply each movement that your partner has performed? Can you see a pattern to the innervation of the different movements?

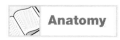 **Anatomy**

▶ Now that you have seen what the nerves can do, study the arrangement of the nerves in the pelvis. Note that the ventral rami of the sacral and coccygeal nerves form the sacral and coccygeal plexuses. The coccygeal plexus is small, so just note the area of skin that is supplied by this and concentrate on the sacral plexus.

▶ Before you do this, look at the contribution of the autonomic nerves to the sacral plexus. You will note that the sympathetic nervous system has a thoracolumbar outflow, but the sympathetic trunk continues downwards into further ganglia in the pelvis, and joins the great plexuses of the pelvis such as the inferior hypogastric plexus, the rectal plexuses, the vesical plexus, the prostatic plexus and the uterovaginal plexus. Note the parasympathetic nerves arising from S2–S4 and passing directly to the pelvic organs via the pelvic splanchnic nerves.

▶ Trace the appearance of the lumbosacral trunk (consisting of part of the ventral ramus of L4 and all of L5) at the medial edge of the psoas muscle and follow it as it descends towards the sacroiliac joint to join the first sacral nerve. Note the position of the sacral plexus in relation to the posterior wall of the pelvic cavity, the piriformis muscle, the internal iliac and superior gluteal blood vessels, the ureter and the colon. Note the formation of the sciatic nerve and its division into:

— Tibial nerve, from the ventral divisions of L4–S3

— Common peroneal nerve, from the dorsal divisions of L4–S2.

▶ For this case, it is not necessary to study the whole of the distribution of the sciatic nerve. Look particularly at the following nerves, tracing their segmental root level of origin, course and distribution:

— Nerve to quadratus femoris and gemellus inferior

— Nerve to obturator internus and gemellus superior

— Nerve to piriformis

— Superior gluteal nerve

— Inferior gluteal nerve

— Posterior femoral cutaneous nerve

— Pudendal nerve

— Pelvic splanchnic nerves

— Muscular branches, to levator ani, coccygeus and sphincter ani internus.

Questions for discussion

■ To which area of the body might pain be referred from:
  – the bladder
  – the uterus
  – the rectum
  – the sacroiliac joint
  – the lumbosacral joint

- the prostate gland
- the testis
- the ovary
- the descending colon
- the anus
- the vagina
- the urethra?

■ Where do you put local anaesthetic if you want to perform a surgical procedure on the vagina without a general anaesthetic?

■ How are the pelvic splanchnic nerves involved in:
- micturition
- defaecation
- penile erection in the male
- engorgement of the clitoris in the female?

■ If a person had a compressive lesion of the cauda equina, what symptoms would you expect?

■ From the information given to you so far in this case, do you think that Mrs Thomas has cauda equina compression?

Examination 1

When you examined Mrs Thomas, she was in obvious pain. She could barely stand, and she found it very difficult to move her trunk. However, she looked generally quite well, and there was no evidence of anaemia, loss of weight, jaundice or cyanosis. Her pulse was 80 per minute and regular, and blood pressure was 160/90 mmHg. There were no abnormalities in the cardiovascular or respiratory systems. Palpation of the abdomen revealed no tenderness, masses or enlarged organs. Straight leg raising was limited slightly to about 75° bilaterally. Neurological examination was a little difficult to perform because of the pain, but there appeared to be no gross motor or sensory deficit. The ankle reflexes were absent, but the other reflexes were present. Plantar reflexes were flexor.

Examination of her spine showed no bony tenderness, even in the thoracic region, but there was loss of lumbar lordosis and marked spasm in the paravertebral muscles. There was very little movement between the individual vertebrae of the lumbar spine.

Questions for discussion

■ Do you think that Mrs Thomas's osteoporosis is contributing to her present problem?

■ What do you think of Mrs Thomas's problem now?

■ Are there any further investigations that you would like to have done at this stage?

■ What would be your immediate management of Mrs Thomas?

Activity 14.10

▶ Go to your local butcher's shop or supermarket and get a long bone from a lamb or cow (you used a long bone in Ch. 10 also, so you may still have a piece of bone left over). If you are a vegetarian, you might not want to do this, so you will just have to do the activity with a book instead.

▶ Look at the bone and note some of its features. There may still be some marrow in the cavity of the bone (see Ch. 10). For this case, study the bone itself. Note its hardness and colour.

▶ Cut across the bone so that you can see the circular cross section of a cylinder.

Note that the bone is composed of two different kinds of tissue. The outer layer is dense and looks a bit like ivory; this is called compact bone. Inside this there is a layer of bone which looks a bit like a sponge: this is in fact called spongy (or cancellous) bone. Although compact bone appears very dense, it is in fact quite porous; the difference between compact and spongy bone is merely related to the size of the spaces within the bone structure. Spongy bone consists of a meshwork of trabeculae of bone; these are in fact laid down in response to stresses encountered by the bone, so that their orientation reflects the direction of the forces.

▶ Look at an X-ray of the hip joint or the foot and you should see the trabecular lines quite clearly.

▶ See if you can find a small hole in the bone quite near to one of the joint surfaces, where the nutrient artery enters the bone to supply it. Note:

— The thin fibrous membrane called the periosteum surrounding the bone

— The end of the bone, with its joint surface covered by firm but elastic articular cartilage.

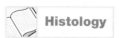 **Histology**

▶ Study the details of bone structure. Note the longitudinally-oriented cylindrical units, termed 'Haversian canals', consisting of a central canal surrounded by concentric rings (lamellae) of bony tissue. Note the bone cells oriented in a concentric fashion with the lamellae, and the presence of blood vessels in the central canal.

Question for discussion

■ What are the functions of bone?

Bone consists of an organic matrix, 90% of which is collagen and 10% of which consists of a number of substances such as:

— Osteocalcin
— Proteoglycans
— Osteonectin
— Sialoproteins.

There are three different types of bone cell:

— Osteoblasts
— Osteoclasts
— Osteocytes.

Note the different origin of osteoblasts and osteoclasts; osteocytes are derived from osteoblasts and are encased in the bone substance. Osteocytes are not inert cells, but communicate with each other via extensions travelling through the canaliculi and may be involved in detecting stresses in the bone.

The main feature of bone is the presence of mineral, in the form of calcium phosphate as hydroxyapatite crystals. This is deposited on the matrix and gives bone its characteristic structure and strength.

Looking at the piece of bone from the butcher, you may be forgiven for thinking that bone is a pretty inert material; in fact, it is very much alive and active.

▶ Have a little light relief with your partner and play the game (I'm not sure whether it has a proper name) where you place your hand on top of your partner's hand, then he places his other hand on top of yours, and finally you place your other hand on top of his. Your partner then takes his bottom hand and places it on top of the 'pile' of hands, you then do the same and the process is repeated as fast as you can do it until one of you makes a mistake. If you think about this for a moment, you will note that although there is a lot of activity going on, the thickness of the 'pile' of hands does not change.

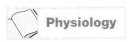 **Physiology**

▶ Look in your textbook; you will see that a similar process occurs in the remodelling of bone.

Bone is continually being formed under the influence of the osteoblast, and is continually being reabsorbed by the osteoclasts. Osteoblasts contain enzymes such as alkaline phosphatase and pyrophosphatase which can prevent the action of inhibitors of mineralisation. Osteoclasts secrete proteolytic enzymes which break down the organic matrix, and acids which cause the bone salts to dissolve. In the normal adult, the rate of bone deposition equals that of resorption so that the total bone mass is approximately constant.

Question for discussion

■ How do you think that osteoblasts and osteoclasts communicate so that bone formation and resorption are linked?

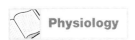 **Physiology**

▶ Study the factors that control the composition of bone. Note that there are a number of hormones that are known to affect bone turnover:
— Vitamin D
— Parathyroid hormone (PTH)
— Calcitonin
— Thyroxine
— Growth hormone
— Somatomedins

— Sex hormones
— Glucocorticoids
— Prostaglandins
— Cytokines
— Osteoclast-stimulating factors.

The first three mentioned have the greatest effects on bone metabolism (see also Ch. 13). As far as bone is concerned, both vitamin D and PTH increase the rate of osteoclastic activity and thus bone resorption, while calcitonin suppresses it.

Questions for discussion

■ How do metastatic deposits of many cancers in bone cause resorption?

■ Bony secondary deposits from cancer of the prostate cause the bone to become sclerotic. How might this happen?

Activity 14.11

▶ Study the development of the most common metabolic bone disease, osteoporosis. This disorder is caused by an excess of bone resorption over production. Note particularly that, although the bone density is reduced, its composition is normal. The loss of bone density occurs with increasing age, but in women it tends to occur at a greater rate. Osteoporosis is only important clinically when it gives rise to fractures, and therefore pain and immobility (which can cause further loss of bone mass).

Questions for discussion

■ Do you think that genetic factors play a part in the development of osteoporosis?

■ Why do you think that women are more likely to develop osteoporosis than men?

■ Which areas are the most common for fractures in people with osteoporosis?

■ How might you prevent the development of osteoporosis?

Bone formation occurs at the periosteal surface, while resorption occurs endosteally. If resorption exceeds formation in a long bone, the thickness of the cortex will be diminished while the diameter will increase. This will lead to loss of bone mass and to weakness.

Questions for discussion

■ What are the radiological features of an osteoporotic spine?

■ How accurate is estimation of bone mass from radiographs?

■ How else may bone mass be measured? How accurate are these methods?

▶ Make a list of the main causes of osteoporosis. Note that:

— The commonest cause is age-related, but increased bone loss may be due to immobility, endocrine causes and a number of other conditions such as rheumatoid arthritis

— The main symptom of osteoporosis is localised pain, with deformity; examination may reveal loss of trunk height, thoracic kyphosis and bone tenderness.

Questions for discussion

■ How does corticosteroid treatment cause osteoporosis?

■ How might immobility cause osteoporosis?

■ What other important conditions may cause bone tenderness?

■ How might you differentiate these causes from osteoporosis?

■ How might you determine the cause of osteoporosis in a patient?

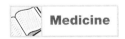 **Medicine**

▶ Study the principles of prevention and treatment of osteoporosis. Note the effect of exercise on bone mass, and the importance of maintaining an adequate calcium and vitamin D intake. Note also the use of hormone replacement therapy in menopausal women, and particularly in young women whose ovaries have been removed at hysterectomy. There have been various other forms of treatment of established osteoporosis, including anabolic steroids, parathyroid hormone, fluoride, calcitonin and biphosphonates.

Questions for discussion

■ What is the effect of oestrogens on bone metabolism?

- Design a research project that would help you determine whether or not hormone replacement therapy was useful in preventing osteoporosis in women undergoing a natural menopause.
- What risks are there in giving oestrogens to postmenopausal women?

Examination 2

You felt that, although Mrs Thomas did have a diagnosis of established osteoporosis, her present problem was not related to this and that there was a mechanical dysfunction in the pelvis. Nevertheless, you avoided any thrust techniques and concentrated on relieving the muscle spasm by stretching and gentle soft tissue manipulation. You also thought that it would be best for her to have a blood test to exclude any underlying serious disorder. With your manual treatment, Mrs Thomas made a speedy recovery, much to the delight and relief of herself and her husband. A week or so later, the blood tests showed the following:

Haemoglobin	13.4 g dl^{-1}
White cell count	$6.8 \times 10^9 \text{ l}^{-1}$
Platelets	$200 \times 10^9 \text{ l}^{-1}$
ESR	15 mm in first hour
Plasma total calcium	2.4 mmol l^{-1}
Plasma phosphate	1.1 mmol l^{-1}
Plasma alkaline phosphatase	240 i.u. l^{-1}

A plain X-ray of Mrs Thomas's lumbar spine and pelvis was reported as normal.

Questions for discussion

- Are any of the blood tests abnormal?
- Do you think that further investigation is required?
- Is your management of Mrs Thomas altered by the results shown?

Discussion

It is very easy to be fooled by a patient's previous diagnosis into assuming that their present problem is related to the same disease process. In the case of Mrs Thomas, her osteoporosis would quite rightly have made you cautious about how you would manage her acute pain. However, the quality of the pain was quite different from her usual ache in the thoracic region, and was located in a different region. One possibility that should occur to you is that of a pathological fracture, sustained when she turned over in bed. This will then raise the possibility of a malignant process destroying the bone. However, the history that she gives you when you visit her is not that of an ill person, and a pathological fracture in the lumbar spine is not all that common without evidence of a disease process going on elsewhere.

Physical examination in Mrs Thomas does not reveal any features of malignant infiltration of bone – there is no anaemia, no bony tenderness and no evidence of a localised primary cancer such as breast or lung.

In a case such as this, it is probably permissible to carry out some gentle soft tissue work to relieve the major symptoms and it is wise to avoid thrust manipulations even if the results of the investigations do not show any specific abnormality. In Mrs Thomas's case, there is good reason to believe that her pain was caused by a mechanical dysfunction of the lower lumbar spine and pelvis, and that this would respond to manual intervention, and this proved to be the case.

Osteoporosis is the most common metabolic bone disease and can also be very difficult to treat. The incidence of fractures of the femoral neck has major financial implications for the health services, particularly in a population which has an increasing number of older people. Symptoms do not appear unless there is collapse of a vertebra or fracture of a long bone. In an individual patient with pain, it is important to exclude causes such as osteomalacia, multiple myeloma and infiltration by leukaemia or metastatic carcinoma, particularly in an older person. The history and physical examination will help to do this, as will some fairly simple investigations. For example, anaemia and a high ESR (or plasma viscosity) may occur in the malignant processes, there will be alterations in plasma calcium and phosphate in osteomalacia, and serum protein analysis will define a monoclonal band in myeloma. In osteoporosis, the blood tests are usually normal, although immobility may cause an increase in the level of calcium in the urine, and bone fracture may increase the blood alkaline phosphatase level.

X-rays in osteoporosis may show reduction of cortical thickness and loss of trabeculae in long bones, and in the vertebrae Schmorl's nodes (protrusion of the intervertebral disc through the end plate). The best radiological sign, however, is collapse of a bone, leading to wedging of the affected vertebrae. Bone scans may show evidence of fracture and may help to exclude secondary malignant deposits; bone density measurements can be made with dual photon absorptiometry to a high degree of accuracy, and are used for research purposes.

The most common cause of osteoporosis is age-related, but it is useful to exclude other causes such as corticosteroid excess and endocrine disease. The most important aspect in the management of osteoporosis is prevention, since treatment of established disease is often unsatisfactory. Calcium intake, exercise, and hormone status in the female with ovarian failure should all be addressed.

FURTHER READING

Barrett-Connor E 1995 The economic and human costs of osteoporotic fracture. American Journal of Medicine 27: 98 (2A): 3S–8S

Lindsay R 1994 Prevention of osteoporosis. Preventative Medicine 23: 722–726

Sambrook P N, Kelly P J, Morrison N A, Eisman J A 1994 Genetics of osteoporosis. British Journal of Rheumatology 33: 1007–1011

Stern P J, Cote P, Dust W 1994 Pelvic insufficiency fracture simulating metastatic bone disease. Journal of Manipulative Physiology and Therapy 17: 485–488

Select bibliography

In addition to the large textbooks of the various subjects, I have found the following books to be helpful. Some of the books are part of a series, and looking at the book given here will direct you to the rest of the series.

Axford J (ed) 1996 Medicine. Blackwell Science, Oxford

Beck E, Francis J L, Souhami R L 1992 Tutorials in differential diagnosis, 3rd edn. Churchill Livingstone, Edinburgh

Burkitt H G, Young B, Health J W (eds) 1993 Wheater's functional histology, 3rd edn. Churchill Livingstone, Edinburgh

Cahill D R (ed) 1997 Lachman's case studies in anatomy, 4th edn. Oxford University Press, Oxford

Cailliet R 1988 Soft tissue pain and disability, 2nd edn. F A Davis, Philadelphia

Chaitow L 1996 Modern neuromuscular techniques. Churchill Livingstone, Edinburgh

Chaitow L 1996 Muscle energy techniques. Churchill Livingstone, Edinburgh

Glass R D 1997 Diagnosis, a brief introduction. Oxford University Press, Oxford

Gross J M, Fetto J, Rose E 1996 Musculoskeletal examination. Blackwell Science, Oxford

Gross R 1996 Psychology, the science of mind and behaviour, 3rd edn. Hodder & Stoughton, London

Kapandji I A 1982 The physiology of the joints. Vol. 1, Upper limb, 5th edn. Churchill Livingstone, Edinburgh

Kapandji I A 1988 The physiology of the joints. Vol. 2, Lower limb, 5th edn. Churchill Livingstone, Edinburgh

Kapandji I A 1982 The physiology of the joints. Vol. 3, Vertebral column. Churchill Livingstone, Edinburgh

Lumley J S P 1990 Surface anatomy: the anatomical basis of clinical examination. Churchill Livingstone, Edinburgh

McConway K (ed) 1994 Studying health and disease. Open University Press, Buckingham

Mackinnon P C B, Morris J F 1986 Oxford textbook of functional anatomy. Vol. 1, Musculoskeletal system. Oxford University Press, Oxford

Mackinnon P C B, Morris J F 1988 Oxford textbook of functional anatomy. Vol. 2, Thorax and abdomen. Oxford University Press, Oxford

Mackinnon P C B, Morris J F 1990 Oxford textbook of functional anatomy. Vol. 3, Head and neck. Oxford University Press, Oxford

McPhee S J, Lingappa V R, Ganong W F, Lange J D 1995 Pathophysiology of disease – an introduction to clinical medicine. Appleton & Lange, Connecticut

Marshall W J 1992 Clinical chemistry, 2nd edn. Gower Medical, London

Moore K L 1992 Clinically oriented anatomy, 3rd edn. Williams & Wilkins, Baltimore

Parums D V (ed) 1996 Essential clinical pathology. Blackwell Science, Oxford

Rang H P, Dale M M, Ritter J M 1995 Pharmacology, 3rd edn. Churchill Livingstone, Edinburgh

Robergs R A, Roberts S O 1997 Exercise physiology. Exercise, performance and clinical applications. Mosby, St Louis

Seale C, Pattison S (eds) 1994 Medical knowledge: doubt and certainty. Open University Press, Buckingham

Souhami R L, Moxham J 1994 Textbook of medicine, 2nd edn. Churchill Livingstone, Edinburgh

Squire L F, Novelline R A 1988 Fundamentals of radiology, 4th edn. Harvard University Press, Cambridge, Mass.

Toghill P J 1995 Examining patients. Edward Arnold, London

Travell J G, Simons D G 1991 Myofascial pain and dysfunction. The trigger point manual, Vol. 1. Williams & Wilkins, Baltimore

Travell J G, Simons D G 1994 Myofascial pain and dysfunction. The trigger point manual, Vol. 2. Williams & Wilkins, Baltimore

Willard F 1993 Medical neuroanatomy – a problem-oriented manual with annotated atlas. J B Lippincott, Philadelphia

Venables G S, Bates D, Cartlidge N E F 1988 Case presentations in neurology. Butterworth Heinemann, Oxford

Index

BELMONT UNIVERSITY LIBRARY

BELMONT UNIVERSITY LIBRARY

DATE RETURN

NOV 0 9 2006			
NOV 0 2 REC'D			